Movement Disorders Rehabilitation

Hsin Fen Chien
Orlando Graziani Povoas Barsottini
Editors

Movement Disorders Rehabilitation

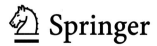 Springer

KH

Editors
Hsin Fen Chien
Department of Neurology
Hospital das Clínicas da Faculdade de
    Medicina da Universidade de São Paulo
São Paulo, Brazil

Department of Orthopedics and
    Traumatology
Faculdade de Medicina da Universidade de
    São Paulo
São Paulo, Brazil

Orlando Graziani Povoas Barsottini
Department of Neurology
Universidade Federal de São Paulo
São Paulo, Brazil

ISBN 978-3-319-46060-4   ISBN 978-3-319-46062-8   (eBook)
DOI 10.1007/978-3-319-46062-8

Library of Congress Control Number: 2016959000

Printed on acid-free paper

This Springer imprint is published by Springer Nature
The registered company is Springer International Publishing AG
The registered company address is: Gewerbestrasse 11, 6330 Cham, Switzerland

4/9/18

To my mother and father (in memoriam)
Love is patient, love is kind. … It always
protects, always trusts, always hopes,
always perseveres. Love never fails.
To my loving and supportive family.

Hsin Fen Chien

To my parents Ruth and Orlando
(in memoriam).

Orlando Barsottini

Foreword

Up until 30 years ago neurologists were typecast as brilliant, austere men who talked with ease about areas of the brain that most other doctors had forgotten existed. They adored diagnosis, many suffered from spanophilia and most had little interest in time-consuming treatments.

Then neurorehabilitation arrived making the more go ahead neurologist realise that there was now a lot to offer patients. Even its more Luddite exponents realised that if they did not start to become more involved in the care of patients with chronic neurological disability, then they faced extinction in both the public and private health care systems.

The notion that external intervention could facilitate the brain's plasticity and potentially reduce the consequences of brain injury was a new exciting concept.

Specialist neurorehabilitation services now play a vital role in the management of patients after their immediate medical and surgical needs have been met, in optimising their recovery and supporting their safe transition back to the community. Modern technology is now increasingly being used to supplement physical and cognitive therapies in restoring function in patients with traumatic brain injury and stroke.

With a few notable exceptions, neurologists with a special interest in the treatment of movement disorders have been slow to embrace neurorehabilitation. Many are sceptical of the "neurobling" of plasticity and functional imaging and look upon the use of complementary approaches to therapy such as tango dancing and Tai Chi with grave suspicion. This resistance to a more holistic treatment approach may in part reflect the fact that abnormal movement disorders rarely present with devastating acute or subacute disability, and that a number of efficacious medical and surgical treatments are available for the commoner disorders. This has led to less engagement with physical and speech therapists in comparison with, say, the field of multiple sclerosis, so that despite the increasing evidence base and intriguing preclinical and clinical science in the neurorehabilitation of movement disorders, sophisticated state-of-the-art facilities are thin on the ground.

This excellent book edited by Chien Hsin Fen and Orlando Barsottini hopefully draws movement disorder and neurorehabilitation specialists into a fascinating and largely untapped fruitful field of research that has the potential to vastly improve the lives of the thousands of people living with the disabilities caused by basal ganglia dysfunction.

The National Hospital, Queen Square   Andrew Lees
London, UK
July 2016

Contents

Contributors

Fereshte Adib Saberi, M.D. Movement Disorders Section, Department of Neurology, Hannover Medical School, Hannover, Germany

Mariana Jardim Azambuja, S.L.P., M.Sc. Department of Neurology, Hospital das Clínicas da Faculdade de Medicina da Universidade de São Paulo, São Paulo, Brazil

Egberto Reis Barbosa, M.D., Ph.D. Department of Neurology, Hospital das Clínicas da Faculdade de Medicina da Universidade de São Paulo, São Paulo, Brazil

Orlando Graziani Povoas Barsottini, M.D., Ph.D. Department of Neurology, Universidade Federal de São Paulo, São Paulo, Brazil

Francisco Cardoso, M.D., Ph.D., F.A.A.N. Movement Disorders Unit, Neurology Service, The Federal University of Minas Gerais, Belo Horizonte, MG, Brazil

Hsin Fen Chien, M.D., Ph.D. Department of Neurology, Hospital das Clínicas da Faculdade de Medicina da Universidade de São Paulo, São Paulo, Brazil

Department of Orthopedics and Traumatology, Faculdade de Medicina da Universidade de São Paulo, São Paulo, Brazil

Juliana Conti, O.T. Department of Neurology, Hospital das Clínicas da Faculdade de Medicina da Universidade de São Paulo, São Paulo, Brazil

Tamine Teixeira da Costa Capato, P.T., M.Sc. Department of Physical Therapy, Hospital das Clínicas da Faculdade de Medicina da Universidade de São Paulo, São Paulo, Brazil

Carolina de Oliveira Souza, P.T., M.Sc. Department of Neurology, Hospital das Clínicas da Faculdade de Medicina da Universidade de São Paulo, São Paulo, Brazil

Giovana Diaferia, S.L.P., M.Sc. Department of Neurology, Universidade Federal de São Paulo, São Paulo, Brazil

Alice Estevo Dias, S.L.P., Ph.D. Department of Neurology, Hospital das Clínicas da Faculdade de Medicina da Universidade de São Paulo, São Paulo, Brazil

Dirk Dressler, M.D., Ph.D. Movement Disorders Section, Department of Neurology, Hannover Medical School, Hannover, Germany

Alberto J. Espay, M.D., M.Sc. Department of Neurology, University of Cincinnati, Cincinnati, OH, USA

Maria Eliza Freitas, M.D. Morton and Gloria Shulman Movement Disorders Centre and the Edmond J. Safra Program in Parkinson's Disease, Toronto Western Hospital, University of Toronto, Toronto, ON, Canada

Greydon Gilmore, M.Sc., B.Sc. Physiology and Pharmacology, Western University, London, ON, Canada

Monica Santoro Haddad, M.D., M.Sc. Department of Neurology, Hospital das Clínicas da Faculdade de Medicina da Universidade São Paulo, São Paulo, Brazil

Mandar Jog, M.D., F.R.C.P.C. Clinical Neurological Sciences, London Health Sciences Centre, London, ON, Canada

Débora Maia, M.D., M.Sc. Movement Disorders Unit, Neurology Service, The Federal University of Minas Gerais, Belo Horizonte, MG, Brazil

Renato P. Munhoz, M.D., Ph.D. Morton and Gloria Shulman Movement Disorders Centre and the Edmond J. Safra Program in Parkinson's Disease, Toronto Western Hospital, University of Toronto, Toronto, ON, Canada

José Luiz Pedroso, M.D., Ph.D. Department of Neurology, Universidade Federal de São Paulo, São Paulo, Brazil

Marcelo Masruha Rodrigues, M.D., Ph.D. Division of Child Neurology, Universidade Federal de São Paulo, São Paulo, Brazil

Hélio A.G. Teive, M.D., Ph.D. Universidade Federal do Paraná, Curitiba, PR, Brazil

Mariana Callil Voos, P.T., Ph.D. Department of Physical Therapy, Faculdade de Medicina da Universidade de São Paulo, São Paulo, Brazil

Marise Bueno Zonta, P.T., Ph.D. Universidade Federal do Paraná, Curitiba, PR, Brazil

Introduction

1

Hsin Fen Chien

Movement Disorders and Rehabilitation

Movement disorders (MD) represent an area of neurological dysfunction based on clinical phenomenology rather than on an anatomical location. The term was coined in 1968 by Stanley Fahn and was quickly adopted by the neurological community.

Movement disorders could be defined as neurological syndromes in which there is either an excess of movement or a paucity of voluntary and automatic movements, unrelated to weakness or spasticity. The former are commonly referred to as hyperkinesia (excessive movements), dyskinesia (unnatural movements), and abnormal involuntary movements. The paucity of movement group is referred to as hypokinesia (decreased amplitude of movement), bradykinesia (slowness of movement) and akinesia (loss of movement) [1].

The key factor for the modern classification of MD is the phenomenology of the movements. The conditions are therefore grouped into two major groups: hyperkinesia (ataxia, athetosis, ballism, chorea, dyskinesia, dystonia, hemifacial spasm, hyperekplexia, myoclonus, tics, tremor, restless legs), and hypokinesia (bradykinesia/parkinsonism, freezing, catatonia).

The list of the diseases is constantly expanding, as does MD as a subspecialty of neurology. A survey conducted by the American Academy of Neurology in 2008 reported that 9 % of the residents going into a fellowship chose MD. Moreover, general internists, family physicians, and neurologists were questioned about three

H.F. Chien, M.D., Ph.D. (✉)
Department of Neurology, Hospital das Clínicas da Faculdade de Medicina da Universidade de São Paulo, São Paulo, Brazil

Department of Orthopedics and Traumatology, Faculdade de Medicina da Universidade de São Paulo, São Paulo, Brazil
e-mail: chien.74@fmusp.org.br

© Springer International Publishing Switzerland 2017
H.F. Chien, O.G.P. Barsottini (eds.), *Movement Disorders Rehabilitation*,
DOI 10.1007/978-3-319-46062-8_1

neurological conditions: transient cerebrovascular events, dementia and Parkinson's disease (PD). For the issue of the transient event, over 50% of internists felt that the primary care physicians should manage the condition alone; for dementia over 70% felt the same. Only for PD was there a majority recommending referral to a MD specialist [2].

Shih et al. [3] surveyed the approximate percentage of diagnoses and conditions seen in movement disorders clinics in North America and the frequency was: PD 51.9%, dystonia 15.1%, tremor 13.7%, ataxia 7.5%, and others MD 10.7%. There is a high frequency of PD in MD clinics worldwide as it is the second most common neurodegenerative disorder after Alzheimer's disease. Because of the combination of the aging process and a chronic condition, it represents an economic burden for the patient and for payers.

According to Kowal et al. [4], the population with PD in the USA incurred medical expenses of approximately $14 billion in 2010. Nursing home care is a major contributor to the medical cost burden, whereas reduced employment is a major indirect cost of PD.

Another study conducted by Johnson et al. [5], demonstrated that slowing disease progression by any disease modification treatment would reduce the symptom burden and be cost-effective. A scenario where PD progressed 20% slower than a hypothetical base case resulted in net monetary benefits of a 25% reduction in excess costs spread over a longer expected survival period.

The burden of chronic conditions such as PD is projected to grow substantially over the next few decades as the size of the elderly population grows. Such projections give impetus to the need for innovative new treatments to prevent, delay onset, or alleviate symptoms of PD and other similar diseases, Kowal et al. [4] concluded.

However, preventing, delaying or alleviating any chronic debilitating condition, which is the case in most MDs, by reducing the cost burden should not be the only goal of any treatment; the quality of life of patients and caregivers should also be improved.

Quality of life (QoL) is defined as "individuals' perception of their position in life in the context of the culture and value systems in which they live and in relation to their goals, expectations, standards and concerns. It is a broad ranging concept acted in a complex way by the persons' physical health, psychological state, level of independence, social relationships and their relationship to salient features of their environment" [6].

Chronic conditions are associated with increased physical impairment, which leads to a reduced positive affect, reduced control/autonomy, and less enjoyment and fulfillment in life [7]. Most MD conditions are chronic and the involuntary movements impair physical functions. In the case of PD, the nondopaminergic motor features, including impairment in gait, postural control, and falls, become the sources of disability [8] and poorer QoL.

A systematic review to identify the demographic and clinical factors that predict the health-related QoL of people with PD concluded that depression, disease severity, and disease disability were found to predict poor quality of life. The motor system that contributed most to overall life quality was gait impairment [9]. Shulman et al. [10] analyzed the evolution of disability in PD and concluded that the period of disability in PD occurs between total Unified Parkinson Disease Rating Scale (UPDRS) 30 and 60, between Hoehn and Yahr (HY) stages II to III, and 3–7 years after diagnosis. The stage of preclinical disability can potentially be targeted by pharmacological and nonpharmacological interventions to delay disability. They also identified that gait impairment was the leading cause of disability in PD.

A quick search in the literature will guide the reader to many research studies showing improvement in PD patients' motor symptoms, including gait, with diverse rehabilitation programs and improvement of their QoL [11]. This is also true for the second most common condition seen in an MD clinic, dystonia. Queiroz et al. [12], carried out a physical therapy program in cervical dystonia patients and observed not only symptomatic improvement of dystonia, but also of their QoL.

According to the World Health Organization, rehabilitation is defined as a set of measures that assist individuals who experience or are likely to experience disability to achieve and maintain optimal functioning in interaction with their environments, is instrumental in enabling people with functional limitations to remain in or return to their home or community, to live independently, and to participate in education, the labor market, and civic life.

Moreover, the rehabilitation measures are aimed at achieving: prevention and slowing the rate of loss of function; improvement or restoration of function; compensation for loss of function; and maintenance of current function.

In other words, rehabilitation of people with disabilities is a process aimed at enabling them to reach and maintain their optimal physical, sensory, intellectual, psychological, and social–functional levels. Rehabilitation provides disabled people with the tools they need to attain independence and self-determination [13].

For the rehabilitation process to be effective and help chronically disabled patients to regain or maintain their functions, the participation of an effective and qualified team is essential [14]. It is not within the scope of this chapter to discuss the advantages or disadvantages of different models of professional teams (multidisciplinary, interdisciplinary or transdisciplinary) and which is advocated for the care of MD patients.

Although the recent literature has provided evidence of the benefits of rehabilitation in MD many points remain unanswered and future studies should address these questions. Most of the clinical trials indicate good results with rehabilitation intervention, but they are of short duration and cannot be translated to measure long-term benefits. The definition of a rehabilitation team is vast and the composition of health-allied professionals varies from study to study. A definition of what constitutes the minimal requirements for a multidisciplinary team for MD trials is needed. There is no consensus in assessment tools to rate rehabilitation interventions in many MD diseases. The dose and frequency of the intervention is also problematic: how much is enough? The environment in which studies are conducted varies from community to outpatient and inpatient settings. Furthermore, different stages of the disease require different rehabilitation strategies and management approaches. Good robust studies should answer these questions.

References

1. Fahn S. Classification of movement disorders. Mov Disord. 2011;26:947–57.
2. Farbman ES. The case for subspecialization in neurology: movement disorders. Front Neurol. 2011;2:22.
3. Shih LC, Tarsy D, Okun MS. The current state and needs of North American movement disorders fellowship programs. Parkinsons Dis. 2013;2013:701426. doi:10.1155/2013/701426.
4. Kowal SL, Dall TM, Chakrabarti R, Storm MV, Jain A. The current and projected economic burden of Parkinson's disease in the United States. Mov Disord. 2013;28:311–18.
5. Johnson SJ, Diener MD, Kaltenboeck A, Birnbaum HG, Siderowf AD. An economic model of Parkinson's disease: implications for slowing progression in the United States. Mov Disord. 2013;28:319–26.
6. The World Health Organization Quality of Life Assessment (WHOQOL): development and general psychometric properties. Soc Sci Med. 1998; 46:1569–85.
7. Sexton E, King-Kallimanis BL, Layte R, Hickey A. CASP-19 special section: how does chronic disease status affect CASP quality of life at older ages? Examining the WHO ICF disability domains as mediators of this relationship. Aging Ment Health. 2015;19:622–33.
8. Rochester L, Espay AJ. Multidisciplinary rehabilitation in Parkinson's disease: a milestone with future challenges. Mov Disord. 2015;30:1011–13.
9. Soh SE, Morris ME, McGinley JL. Determinants of health-related quality of life in Parkinson's disease: a systematic review. Parkinsonism Relat Disord. 2011;17:1–9.
10. Shulman LM, Gruber-Baldini AL, Anderson KE, Vaughan CG, Reich SG, Fishman PS, Weiner WJ. The evolution of disability in Parkinson disease. Mov Disord. 2008;23:790–6.
11. Monticone M, Ambrosini E, Laurini A, Rocca B, Foti C. In-patient multidisciplinary rehabilitation for Parkinson's disease: a randomized controlled trial. Mov Disord. 2015;30:1050–8.
12. Queiroz MA, Chien HF, Sekeff-Sallem FA, Barbosa ER. Physical therapy program for cervical dystonia: a study of 20 cases. Funct Neurol. 2012;27:187–92.
13. WHO Guidelines on Health-Related Rehabilitation (Rehabilitation Guidelines). 2016. http://who.int/disabilities/care/rehabilitation_guidelines_concept.pdf. Accessed 27 Mar 2016.
14. Shortell SM, Marsteller JA, Lin M, Pearson ML, Wu SY, Mendel P, et al. The role of perceived team effectiveness in improving chronic illness care. Med Care. 2004;42:1040–8.

Parkinson's Disease

2

Hsin Fen Chien, Egberto Reis Barbosa,
Carolina de Oliveira Souza, Alice Estevo Dias,
and Juliana Conti

Overview of Parkinson's Disease

Introduction

Parkinson's disease is the second most common neurodegenerative disorder worldwide and its prevalence ranges from 18 to 418 cases per 100,000 of the population and 102–190 per 100,000 in Western countries [1]. It affects both men and women, but is a little more common in men.

The disease typically develops after the age of 50 and may affect up to 2 % of the population older than 65 years. The projection of number of people with PD will double in 2050 because the population is aging [2]. Early-onset PD denotes onset of the disease below the age of 40 years and juvenile PD when the age is below 21 years.

H.F. Chien, M.D., Ph.D.
Department of Neurology, Hospital das Clínicas da Faculdade de Medicina da Universidade de São Paulo, São Paulo, Brazil

Department of Orthopedics and Traumatology, Faculdade de Medicina da Universidade de São Paulo, São Paulo, Brazil
e-mail: chien.74@fmusp.org.br

E.R. Barbosa, M.D., Ph.D. (✉) • C. de Oliveira Souza, P.T., M.Sc. • A.E. Dias, S.L.P., Ph.D.
J. Conti, O.T.
Department of Neurology, Hospital das Clínicas da Faculdade de Medicina da Universidade de São Paulo, São Paulo, Brazil
e-mail: egbertob@8415.com.br; souzaco@ig.com.br; alice.estevo@gmail.com

© Springer International Publishing Switzerland 2017
H.F. Chien, O.G.P. Barsottini (eds.), *Movement Disorders Rehabilitation*,
DOI 10.1007/978-3-319-46062-8_2

Pathological Features

The anatomopathological abnormalities of PD are characterized by neuronal loss and intraneuronal inclusions known as Lewy bodies [3]. These cytoplasmic eosinophilic inclusions are composed of free and ubiquitin-conjugated proteins, enzymes, and cytoskeletal proteins. The proteinaceous material includes neurofilament protein, ubiquitin, and alpha-synuclein (AS). The core consists of aggregates of ubiquitin-conjugated protein and the halo of neurofilament protein and alpha-synuclein.

It is believed that the degeneration process begins decades before the first motor signs appear. Lesions initially occur in Auerbach's and Meissner's myenteric plexuses, olfactory bulb, and the lower brain stem. Thereafter, the substantia nigra (SN), basal prosencephalic nuclei, and the limbic system are affected. Lewy bodies are found in cortical association areas in later stages of the disease [4]. In the prodromal phase, or pre-motor stage, symptoms such as hyposmia, gastrointestinal dysfunction, depression, and sleep disturbances (i.e., rapid eye movement [REM]) may be the initial features of the disease.

Etiopathogenesis

The etiology of PD is not fully understood, it is likely that there is a complex interaction of environmental, genetic, and physiological factors, such as the aging process. The evidence for the environmental influences is derived from case reports of parkinsonism due to exposure to toxic agents, neurotoxin-induced parkinsonism in animal models, and epidemiological studies on risk factors for PD.

Van Maele-Fabry et al. [5], systematically reviewed cohort studies and verified that occupational exposure to pesticides increases the risk of PD. The main toxic compounds related to PD are heavy metals (e.g., manganese), pesticides (e.g., rotenone), and herbicides (e.g., paraquat).

On the other hand, regular coffee intake and smoking reduce the risk of PD. More than 50 studies have consistently demonstrated that smokers are less likely to develop the disease than people who never smoked and some studies suggest that nicotine may be neuroprotective. However, in patients in whom PD has already been diagnosed, disease progression is not affected by cigarette smoking [6, 7]. Caffeine blocks adenosine A2A receptors that are highly expressed in the basal ganglia circuitry, especially in the striatum. Istradefylline, an adenosine A2A receptor blocker, has a symptomatic effect on PD patients and is possibly a neuroprotector [8].

Recently, a theory has been proposed linking the protective effect of smoking and coffee consumption and the hypothesis of the gut as the origin of PD. According to the researchers, both cigarettes and coffee may induce changes in the composition of microbiota, with a shift toward a more anti-inflammatory state, which lessens the formation of misfolded alpha-synuclein in enteric nerves [9].

Our knowledge regarding the genetic basis of PD has increased remarkably since the identification of the first gene causing PD (*SNCA*, formerly *PARK1*) by

Polymeropoulos et al. [10]. The causative genes have not yet been established for the 20 loci hitherto related to PD. These loci have been identified by genetic linkage analysis in large families or genome-wide association studies on a population. Some mutations confer higher susceptibility to the development of the disease, but the study of monogenic forms led to the identification of genes causing either autosomal dominant (*SNCA*, *LRRK2*, *VPS35*), or autosomal recessive (*PARK2*, *DJ1*, *PINK1*, *ATP13A2*) familial PD.

Ageing is an important risk factor for developing PD and it can be observed in epidemiological data. The disease occurs infrequently under the age of 40, but affects over 1 % of population after 60 years of age and rises to 5 % of the population over 85 [11].

The degeneration of SN pars compacta neurons is irreversible and results in the reduction of dopamine production, leading to functional abnormalities in the basal nucleus pathways. Neuropathological studies indicate that the rate of neuronal loss in the SN ranges between 5 and 10 % for each decade [12, 13]. The proportion of neuronal fallout is much higher than what is observed in neocortical neurons, which is approximately 10 % over the entire life span [14].

After the discovery of alpha-synuclein as the primary structural component of Lewy bodies, researchers have focused on understanding its role in mechanisms underlying neuronal death. It is assumed that an imbalance between the aggregation of AS and its clearance, via the ubiquitin proteasome pathway or autophagy, can result in accumulation of oligomers, protofibrils, and fibrils [15]. These aggregates, which may be toxic, interfere in critical cellular functions, particularly mitochondrial activity and axonal transport.

Moreover, it is important to mention the identification of toxic AS being eliminated from the neurons via unusual secretory mechanisms. These extracellular AS can disseminate to others neurons or glial cells and trigger intracellular aggregations that promote the neurodegenerative process. This conjecture derived from the postmortem analysis of brain from PD patients who had undergone brain tissue transplantation. Accumulation of AS and Lewy bodies were found in previous unremarkable fetal grafted neurons [16]. These findings have raised the hypothesis that AS propagation might behave as a prion-like disease.

There is a large body of evidence suggesting that mitochondrial dysfunction plays a central role in the etiopathogenesis of PD. The neurotoxins rotenone and 1-methyl-4-phenyl-1,2,3,6-tetrahydropyridine (MPTP) induce parkinsonism by inhibiting the mitochondrial complex I electron transport chain. Several PD-associated genes interface with pathways regulating mitochondrial function [17] or in mitophagy, which is the specific and selective targeted removal of excess or damaged mitochondria from the cell via autophagy.

Recently, inflammation has become implicated as a major pathogenic factor in the onset and progression of Parkinson's disease [18]. Reactive microgliosis, T cell infiltration, and increased expression of inflammatory cytokines are prominent features of the inflammatory process [19]. Recent reports indicate that accumulated aggregated AS can be actively secreted or released by dying neurons to the extracellular space; extracellular AS in turn activates surrounding astrocytes and microglia, eliciting glial pro-inflammatory activity.

Clinical Manifestation

Four motor symptoms are considered cardinal in PD: resting tremor, rigidity, brady-kinesia, and postural instability. For the diagnosis of parkinsonian syndrome, the presence of bradykinesia is necessary in association with one of the other three symptoms to ascertain nigrostriatal dopaminergic pathway degeneration.

Bradykinesia is a motor abnormality characterized by a lack of movement and a slowness in the initiation and execution of voluntary and automatic movements associated with difficulty in changing motor patterns, in the absence of motor weakness. This motor dysfunction may also encompass the decrement of repetitive movements, fatigue, and problems in performing more than one task at the same time. Patients also suffer a decline in their fine motor skills, which can lead to difficulties with buttoning clothes, brushing teeth, cutting food, writing or typing on the computer keyboard.

Other motor abnormalities related to bradykinesia are reduced facial expression (hypomimia), body gestures, and automatic swallowing reflex; this last results in excessive saliva in the mouth and drooling (sialorrhea). The gait is characterized by small quick steps and a reduced arm swing. Patients may also have trouble initiating or continuing movement (freezing), and quickening their normal stride (festination). The typical configuration of speech changes associated with bradykinesia (phonation, resonance, articulation, and prosody) is known as hypokinetic dysarthria.

Rigidity is one of the major signs of PD and is characterized by increased stiffness experienced during passive mobilization of a limb, which remains in the position that has been imposed after stretching and for this reason is termed plastic hypertonia. The hypertonia can be constant or intermittent (cogwheel phenomenon). It affects preferentially the flexor muscles leading to a classical abnormal posture (simian) with flexion of the hips and knees.

Parkinson's tremor is clinically characterized by a resting tremor, which enhances when walking and during mental stress, diminishes by voluntary Parkinson's disease (PD) clinical manifestation movement of the affected body part, and disappears during sleep. It occurs at frequency between 4 and 6 Hz and predominantly affects the hands, progressing to forearm pronation/supination.

Postural instability is associated with increased falls and loss of independence. Many factors contribute to balance impairment, including disturbed postural reflexes and poor voluntary movement control. It can be present at diagnosis, but becomes more prevalent and worsens with disease progression [20].

Nonmotor symptoms in PD are common and affect cognition, behavior, sleep, autonomic function, and sensory function. Mild cognitive changes may be present at the time of diagnosis or even early in the course of the disease. Approximately 15–20 % of patients develop dementia in the advanced phase of PD. The patients may experience depression at any stage of the disease and its prevalence in PD is about 40 %. Autonomic symptoms in PD can include constipation, pain, genitourinary problems, and orthostatic hypotension.

Diagnosis

The diagnosis of PD relies mainly upon medical history and neurological examination and tests are ordered to rule out other conditions. The hallmarks for improving diagnostic accuracy in PD are: (a) absence of atypical parkinsonism (early severe autonomic involvement, early severe dementia, Babinski sign, supranuclear gaze palsy, neuroleptic treatment at onset of symptoms, history of repeated strokes, and history recent encephalitis) and (b) unilateral onset [21, 22].

Differential Diagnosis

The Parkinsonian syndrome encompasses neurological conditions other than PD, and it can be grouped as secondary parkinsonism and degenerative atypical parkinsonism.

Drug-induced parkinsonism (DIP) is the most common etiology of secondary parkinsonism. These substances block central nerve system D1 and D2 dopamine receptors highly expressed in the striatum, where most of the nigral dopaminergic projections are found. The most common drug related to DIP is neuroleptic, with the exception of clozapine, which displays a high affinity for the dopamine D4 receptor, which in turn has a low density in the human striatum. Many other medications are known to produce DIP: calcium channel blockers, gastrointestinal prokinetics (antiemetics), and dopamine-depleting drugs. The symptoms usually resolve within weeks to months after stopping the offending drug.

Other causes of secondary parkinsonism may be identified properly by anamnesis and laboratory tests. MRI is also used to identify features that may indicate secondary parkinsonism such as normal pressure hydrocephalus, brain tumor, and basal ganglia calcification.

Atypical parkinsonism or Parkinson-plus are terms used to describe syndromes that share features similar to PD (usually akinesia and rigidity), but are different conditions. Frequently associated symptoms are dysautonomia, cerebellar signs, pyramidal tract signs, and ocular signs. The presentation is usually symmetrical and the patients respond poorly to antiparkinsonian drugs. Parkinson-plus syndromes can be broadly grouped into two types: synucleinopathies and tauopathies. Clinically, the most common forms of atypical parkinsonism are as follows: multiple system atrophy (MSA), progressive supranuclear palsy (PSP), corticobasal ganglionic degeneration (CBD), and dementia with Lewy bodies (DLB).

A good response to antiparkinsonian drugs supports the diagnosis of PD, although up to 20 % of PSP [23] and 50 % of MSA patients [24] initially have a good response to levodopa. Particularly in MSA, some patients maintain a response throughout the course of the illness.

Parkinson's disease has a slow progression and the patients are usually independent in the first 5 years after the diagnosis. Rapidly evolving parkinsonism or disability raise a high degree of suspicion for atypical parkinsonism. Levodopa-induced dyskinesia development after a long and sustained response to levodopa is indicative of idiopathic PD.

Neuroimaging techniques (computed tomography and magnetic resonance imaging [MRI]), single photon emission computed tomography (SPECT), and positron emission tomography (PET) are useful for differentiating PD from other parkinsonian disorders. These functional techniques use different radiotracers to measure dopaminergic function in the basal ganglia and can be indicated for supportive diagnostic aid [25].

Transcranial ultrasound detects ultrasound echoes from the brain structures. About 90 % of patients with clinically established PD were reported to show bilaterally increased echogenicity from the lateral midbrain [26]. Although it is a promising technique, increased echogenicity was reported in 10 % of healthy individuals.

Olfactory dysfunction is an early feature of PD and a smelling test may aid in the early diagnosis of this disorder. Olfactory dysfunction often precedes the onset of the cardinal motor symptoms of PD by several years. The testing can be a supportive diagnostic tool in differentiating PD from other parkinsonian disorders or essential tremor [27].

Diffusion-weighted imaging (DWI), a different MRI technique, has been used for the differential diagnosis of PD and MSA. DWI is commonly used to determine the random movement of water molecules that are aligned with fiber tracts in the central nervous system. Quantification of diffusion is possible by applying field gradients of different degrees of diffusion sensitization. DWI enables the assessment of the water's apparent diffusion coefficient (ADC), a measure of tissue water diffusivity, and may detect changes in the microstructural integrity of nervous tissue earlier than conventional T1- or T2-weighted MRI [28, 29].

The loss of SN dopaminergic neurones, which is most prominent in sub-regions called nigrosomes, is the hallmark of PD. The largest nigrosome of the five nigrosomes described is labeled nigrosome-1 and positioned in the caudal and mediolateral SN. Schwarz et al. [30], demonstrated that healthy nigrosome-1 can be readily depicted on high-resolution 3 T-susceptibility-weighted (SW)-MRI, giving rise to a "swallow tail" appearance of the dorsolateral substantia nigra, and this feature is lost in PD. Therefore, assessing the substantia nigra on SW-MRI for the typical swallow tail appearance has the potential to become a new applicable diagnostic tool for nigral degeneration in PD.

Recently, Al-Bachari et al. [31] utilized a novel MRI technique, including arterial spin labeling (ASL) quantification of cerebral perfusion, and identified altered neurovascular status in PD. The authors hypothesized that disturbance of the neurovascular unit function, which is a complex, metabolically active system of endothelial cells and glial cells in close proximity to a neuron, is altered in the neurodegeneration process leading to their findings.

Symptomatic Management

Levodopa

Levodopa is the most effective drug for the treatment of symptoms of PD. In the 1970s, the advantages of adding a dopa decarboxylase inhibitor to treatment, to reduce the peripheral metabolism of levodopa, were discovered to reduce side effects and gain better symptom control. Treatment with levodopa contributes to greater activity levels, independence, employability, and consequently improvement in the patient's quality of life (QoL) [32, 33].

Long-Term Motor Complications of Levodopa Treatment

Levodopa preparations lead in the long term to the development of motor complications. These comprise abnormal involuntary movements such as dyskinesia and dystonia, along with response fluctuations. Dyskinesia are classified according to their temporal profile after drug administration, namely peak-dose dyskinesia (mainly choreic movements), biphasic dyskinesia, onset and end-of-dose dyskinesia (mainly dystonic and ballistic movements), and finally "off"-period dyskinesia (dystonic movements). Motor fluctuations comprise wearing off, the on–off phenomenon, and freezing.

The pathogenesis of motor complications associated with chronic levodopa therapy is not fully understood. Some of the theories include: presynaptic neuronal degeneration leading to insufficient buffering of released levodopa, postsynaptic changes in dopamine receptor sensitivity and number, partially caused by presynaptic changes, and pharmacokinetic and pharmacodynamic change in chronic dopaminergic therapy [34, 35].

Catechol-O-methyl Transferase Inhibitors

When peripheral decarboxylation is blocked by carbidopa or benserazide, the main metabolic pathway of levodopa is O-methylation by catechol-O-methyltransferase (COMT). COMT inhibitors improve the bioavailability and decrease the elimination of levodopa, and inhibit the formation of 3-O-methyldopa.

Entacapone inhibits COMT peripherally and tolcapone inhibits it centrally and peripherally. These drugs prolong the antiparkinsonian effect of the levodopa and also allow reduction of the dose. The combination of COMT inhibitors and levodopa is indicated in patients with wearing off.

Dopamine Agonists

Dopamine agonists (DAs) work by directly stimulating dopamine receptors in the brain. There are two subclasses of DA: ergoline and non-ergoline agonists. Ergoline dopamine agonists include bromocriptine, pergolide, lisuride, and cabergoline, whereas ropinirole, rotigotine, and pramipexole are non-ergoline agonists. Apomorphine was the first DA shown to improved PD symptoms, but has to be administered subcutaneously.

Dopamine agonists have been used as a monotherapy in de novo patients with the intention of delaying treatment with levodopa. They are also used as an adjunct to levodopa treatment in patients exhibiting motor fluctuation. The use of DA rather than levodopa appears to postpone the onset of motor complications and dyskinesia. Motor complications may be related to the pulsatile use of levodopa, which leads to an imbalance of basal ganglia opioid concentrations and the resetting of voltage gated channels in N-methyl-D-aspartate (NMDA) receptors. Meanwhile, DAs have a longer half-life and differences in receptor selectivity.

Anticholinergics

The oldest class of medicines for treating PD is the anticholinergic (ACH) drugs. Biperiden and trihexyphenidyl reduces cholinergic activity contributing to reestablishing the balance between cholinergic and dopaminergic activity in the striatum. The most recognized use of ACHs is for treating tremors in early or young onset PD, but they do not significantly affect bradykinesia or rigidity. The most common side effects of ACHs include dry mouth, blurred vision, constipation, and difficulty emptying the bladder. Geriatric patients may react with confusional states or develop delirium.

Amantadine

Amantadine, originally used as an antiviral drug, was coincidentally realized to be a treatment for PD, despite being a weak therapy. The drug increases dopamine release and blocks dopamine reuptake. Recent studies have demonstrated it to be a weak antagonist of the NMDA glutamate receptor. Thus, amantadine can influence glutamatergic neurotransmission at corticostriatal synapse or at the subthalamic–internal pallidal synaptic level. Moreover, recent randomized clinical trials have also shown that amantadine reduces dyskinesia and motor fluctuations in patients receiving levodopa [32].

Disease-Modifying Drugs (Neuroprotection)

The two potentially disease-modifying drugs available are selegiline and rasagiline. Both are selective and irreversible monoamine oxidase B (MAO B) propargylamine inhibitors.

Selegiline undergoes hepatic metabolism and the major plasma metabolites are L-methamphetamine, amphetamine, and desmethyl-selegiline. The resultant amphetamines may cause side effects such as: blood pressure oscillations, arrhythmia, and insomnia.

The neuroprotective effect of selegiline was observed in studies with drug-naïve early PD patients. Compared with placebo, selegiline delayed the need for PD symptomatic therapy. However, given the symptomatic effect of selegiline, conclusions could not be drawn regarding the disease-modifying effect of the drug. The symptomatic effect of the MAO B inhibitor in PD is attributed to its ability to prolong the duration of action of both endogenously and exogenously derived dopamine. It is especially indicated for the initial phase of PD treatment and the recommended dose is 10 mg/day.

Rasagiline is a second-generation MAO B inhibitor for the treatment of PD. The recommended dose is 1 mg/day. Unlike selegiline, rasagiline metabolites have no amphetamine-like characteristics, which results in a safer profile and fewer adverse effects [34]. The FDA rejected the granted status "to slow the clinical progression of PD" for rasagiline as sensitivity analyses did not support a disease-modifying benefit. As a result, the FDA has approved it only as a therapy for PD [36]. The drug's symptomatic effect has been proven in monotherapy or in association with levodopa [37].

Surgery

Deep brain stimulation (DBS) is the neurosurgical procedure for the treatment of levodopa-related motor complications. The overall motor effect of subthalamic nucleus stimulation is quantitatively comparable with that obtained with levodopa, but without fluctuations and allows the reduction of dopaminergic medication, secondarily relieving the dyskinesia.

Traditionally, patients with PD are usually referred for DBS 10–15 years after the onset of the disease. However, Schüepbach et al. [38] conducted a trial with PD patients and early motor complications (mean duration of disease, 7.5 years) in which they underwent either neurostimulation plus medical therapy or medical therapy alone. Neurostimulation was superior to medical therapy with regard to motor disability, activities of daily living (ADLs), levodopa-induced motor complications, and time with good mobility and no dyskinesia.

Most clinical studies have excluded older patients (>75 years) from surgery. Nevertheless, DeLong et al. [39] performed a large retrospective cohort study and examined 1,757 individuals who underwent DBS for PD. Patients older than 75 years of age who had DBS surgery showed a similar 90-day complication risk to their younger counterparts. The authors concluded that age alone should not be a primary exclusion criterion for determining candidacy for DBS.

Physical Therapy in Parkinson's Disease

Introduction

Physical therapy (PT) is indicated as adjuvant treatment in PD because most of the motor deficits that lead to loss of independence, falls, and inactivity are difficult to treat with medications and surgery. The number of PT studies in PD has increased considerably in the last few decades, and there is growing evidence that rehabilitation programs (physical, speech and occupational therapy) are effective in improving motor deficits, QoL, and activities of daily living [40].

Many important studies allowed the elaboration of guidelines for evidence-based clinical practice [41–43]. According to Keus et al. [41], the six specific core areas for PT in PD are: (1) gait, (2) balance and falls; (3) posture; (4) transfers; (5) manual activities; (6) physical capacity (exercise). When designing a rehabilitative program for PD, exercise should be "goal-based," that is, aimed at practicing and learning specific activities in the core areas that are impaired (for instance, balance and gait control), thus leading to improved performance in ADLs. It should be considered that the main goals of physiotherapy for PD are person-specific and linked to the stage of disease progression, thus requiring an accurate physical examination and specific measurement tools (Fig. 2.1).

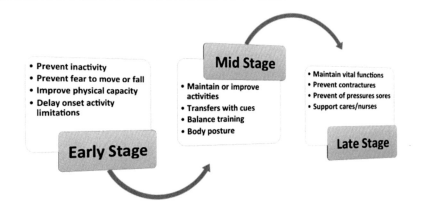

Fig. 2.1 Treatment model for Parkinson's disease (PD; adapted from Keus et al. [42])

Specific Issues in Physiotherapy for PD (Cues)

In 2000, Morris described the theoretical framework supporting the use of PT in PD. The model was based on the pathophysiology of movement disorders in basal ganglia disease, on scientific evidence, and on personal observations of PT interventions in PD. Morris described task-specific strategies for improving the performance of activities (e.g., gait, turning in bed, manual activities, and transfers such as sitting down), the prevention of falls, and the maintenance of physical capacity (e.g., muscle force and aerobic capacity). These strategies incorporate the use of external cues and cognitive movement strategies.

External cues include visual, auditory, or proprioceptive stimuli that are either presented rhythmically or serially (to improve the continuation of gait) or as isolated "one-off" cues (to initiate movements such as gait or transfers). By applying external stimuli instead of the usual internal cues (which normally happens in the healthy brain), alternative circuitries in the brain can be engaged to accomplish the task, while avoiding the defective basal ganglia circuitry [44].

With cognitive movement strategies, complex movements are broken down into separate components. Subjects are trained to perform each of the components separately, and to pay conscious attention to their execution. Mental rehearsing is part of this training. Cognitive movement strategies are mainly used to improve the performance of complex movements such as transfers or manual activities. Morris also stressed the importance of involving the caregiver to optimize therapy.

Goodwin et al. [45], in a systematic review reported the results of PT interventions in patients with PD. The majority of the studies showed that the PT was beneficial for the improvement of functionality, QoL, muscular strength, gait velocity, and balance. Keus et al. [41] reinforce that PT treatment should be based on the following recommendations: (1) external cue strategies; (2) cognitive strategies for movement, in which complex movements are divided into simple subcomponents to be memorized by the patients and executed in a specific order, under conscious control—before the execution of a task, the patient should be guided to practice it mentally (with the objective of overcoming the deficits of sequential movement automatization caused by disorders of the basal ganglia); and (3) balance and gait training with dual tasks and memorized cues. The PT approach to gait and balance disorders in PD has attracted the attention of the scientific community and health professionals over the last few years, because it is known that these disorders are determinants of the decrease in QoL and increase in mortality [46].

The beneficial effects of external cues in the improvement of gait and the decrease in freezing of gait (FOG) episodes are well established in the literature [47]. People with PD could benefit from external cues that are largely used to compensate for the deficiency of the basal ganglia in selected cases and trigger internally learned motor programs [48]. External cues act as potential facilitators of cognitive gait control by selective attention and increase the gait prioritization, mainly during the performance of complex tasks [49, 50]. For example, using a metronome or "clapping hands" to the rhythm of the steps or, taping horizontal lines on the floor that the patient must cross at each step passage.

Cueing via Devices

The use of portable cueing devices has proven effective for the rehabilitation of gait disorders in patients with PD. These devices are currently being developed, incorporating new technologies. Walking sticks [51] and rolling walkers [52] projecting a laser line on the floor have shown efficacy in overcoming FOG and reducing falls in some but not all patients [51].

Light-emitting diodes (LEDs) [53] and auditory devices incorporated into glasses are effective in improving gait parameters in laboratory settings [54]. The studies showed that even with the low serum level of levodopa, some patients could use visual and auditory cues to perform large stride lengths and increase gait velocity. Eyeglasses combining auditory–visual cueing are also effective on gait in advanced PD. Souza et al. [55], used the device in 18 patients who received subthalamic nucleus DBS and gait improvement was observed in the cued condition. These devices hold great promise for becoming personalized, patient-tailored neurorehabilitation assistants in PD (Fig. 2.2).

Gait

Dual Task Training of Gait and Cognition

Many studies address the influence of the cognitive process on posture and gait control. In the last decade the relationship between gait and cognitive functions has received more attention from researchers [56, 57]. In fact, there are cognitive components in the generalization and maintenance of a consistent and normal pattern of gait [58]. The cognitive deficiencies, particularly the executive functions in patients with PD, contribute to the decline in functionality [59–61]. Executive functions such as attention, memory, decision-making, self-perception, and response monitoring are fundamental to the performance of effective daily motor tasks [62].

Fig. 2.2 Auditory and
visual cueing device

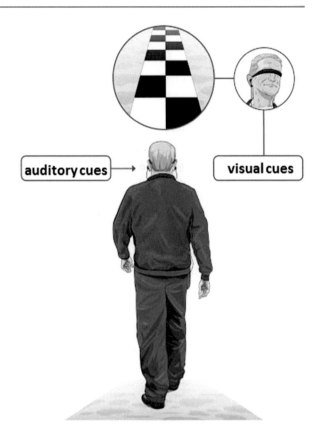

Fig. 2.2 Auditory and
visual cueing device

The correlation between the cognitive decline and gait disorders become more obvious with the progression of PD, leading to a significant impact on the long-term prognosis [63].

It is worth noting that the gait and cognitive relationship is not exclusive to PD patients, also being found in healthy elderly people (even in the early stages of aging) who show subtle cognitive deficiencies that are not detectable by global scales of cognitive tracking. Deficiencies of declarative memory, for example, are associated with the loss of dopamine in the healthy elderly [64].

From this context, challenged training is proposed with the purpose of verifying whether specific motor and cognitive skills could be concomitantly trained. Some authors advocate the need for dual-task training [50, 65] because of the loss of motor performance that requires shared attention with other motor [66, 67] or cognitive tasks [68]. Cognitive tasks are frequently performed during gait in many daily contexts, which justifies the facts that (1) training programs should be designed with the purpose of improving motor and cognitive aspects of dual-task training [69], (2) people with subtle cognitive alterations could benefit from cognitive rehabilitation strategies that involve processes such as planning, initiation, and self-monitoring

[70], (3) patients with better cognitive skills could be highly motivated to engage in a training program [71], yet the kind and severity of cognitive alterations could limit the cognitive skills to compensate for gait abnormalities [72].

Therefore, it could be suggested that a complex training program with motor and cognitive components could be more effective at improving the performance of the dual tasks in a functional gait than a program focused exclusively on the motor function [73]. Motor-cognitive approaches would act as a way to facilitate mechanisms involved in the cognitive reserve. The model of the cognitive reserve postulates the existence of specific experiences and behaviors, which confer protection against the loss related to aging [74].

Posture, Balance and Falls

People with PD demonstrate impaired postural responses. Impairments include hypometric force production, difficulty modifying and scaling postural responses based on the initial context and poor use of the hip strategy [75]. Abnormal proprioceptive–motor integration also contributes to impaired feet-in-place (feet are stationary, no step is performed) postural responses. People with PD tend to over-estimate the size and strength of their movements; even though they may perceive that they are moving with appropriate size and strength, they actually demonstrate hypometric movements and do not reach far enough, walk far enough, or step far enough toward a target when performing without visual feedback [76–78]. Postural instability and falls increase the morbidity and mortality in patients with PD [79]. Early recognition of balance impairments and falls risk contribute to a tailored rehabilitation program, which can minimize complications [80].

Postural adjustments are adaptive responses that maintain postural control. They can be evaluated using static and dynamic posturography, which consists of measuring forces exerted against the ground. Posturography has not only experimental but also clinical relevance, because it can quantify balance disorders, especially in individuals with PD [81–84]. Static posturography assesses body sway under quiet stance tasks. It usually quantifies the center of foot pressure displacements performed on eyes open, eyes closed and dual-task conditions [83, 84]. Dynamic posturography provides data on voluntary motor control, while patients perform tasks or stand still on a platform with external perturbations. It involves latencies of postural responses and body sway mechanisms [81, 85, 86]. Studies approaching PD balance have shown conflicting results; some found increased body sway [87, 88] or no differences in body sway between healthy controls and patients [87]. Others found a reduced or normal sway with a poor correlation with clinical balance tests [89]. These conflicting results stemmed from differences in disease severity, levodopa treatment conditions, and methods of postural instability quantification. In dynamic assessments, most studies evaluated postural control with moving or unstable platforms to observe the responses to external perturbations [86].

In clinical practice, balance tests are used for assessing functional mobility and postural instability in patients with PD. The Movement Disorder Society

(MDS)-commissioned task force [90] assessed the clinimetric properties of existing rating scales, questionnaires, and timed tests that assess posture, gait, and balance in PD and made recommendations on their utilization and the need for modifications or replacement. A literature review was conducted. Identified instruments were evaluated systematically and classified as "recommended," "suggested," or "listed." Inclusion of rating scales was restricted to those that could be readily used in clinical research and practice. The results of their findings were: one rating scale was classified as "recommended" (the UPDRS-derived Postural Instability and Gait Difficulty Score) and two as "suggested" (Tinetti Balance Scale, Rating Scale for Gait Evaluation). Three scales requiring equipment (Berg Balance Scale, Mini-BESTest, Dynamic Gait Index) also fulfilled the criteria for "recommended" and two for "suggested" (FOG score, Gait and Balance Scale). Four questionnaires were "recommended" (Freezing of Gait Questionnaire, Activities-specific Balance Confidence Scale, Falls Efficacy Scale, Survey of Activities, and Fear of Falling in the Elderly–Modified) and four tests were classified as "recommended" (6-min and 10-m walk tests, Timed Up-and-Go, Functional Reach).

Bloem et al. [90], identified several questionnaires that adequately assess FOG and balance confidence in PD and a number of useful clinical tests. However, they found no scale suitable for all clinical purposes to assess gait, balance, and posture, as none of the instruments adequately and separately assesses all constructs, that is, gait (including FOG), balance, and posture. It is also unlikely that a single unidimensional scale can be developed for all three constructs (gait, balance, and posture) because of the potential heterogeneity in the underlying pathophysiology. Given that these concepts are interrelated but independent constructs, it is recommended to assess them simultaneously, but to ensure that separate scores are obtained for the constructs. An ideal future scale should therefore include separate sections for gait, balance, and posture and should specifically address FOG and fear of falling.

Educational status should be taken into consideration when assessing balance, because both executive function and educational level influence balance tests in older adults [91]. People with fewer years of formal education have more difficulty choosing adequate motor strategies for performing tasks. Meanwhile, individuals with higher education, because of their more efficient synaptic and neural networks, may find better motor solutions to imposed motor difficulties. Souza et al. [92] evaluated executive function and functional balance (assessed by the Berg Balance Scale [BBS]) in PD patients (HY score between 2 and 3) and healthy elderly people. Each group of participants was divided by educational status: low (4–10 years of education) or high (11 years or more). The participants with PD and a high educational status performed better on the BBS than did those with PD and low educational status.

The PT program should involve muscle resistance training for quadriceps, hamstrings, and foot extensors to improve posture, muscle stiffness in addition to gait and balance parameters [93, 94]. In PD, there is an imbalance between agonist muscles that facilitate opening movements (e.g., extensors, supinator muscles, external rotators, scapula, and pelvic abductors) and antagonist muscles that facilitate closing movements (flexors, pronators, internal rotators, and adductors), as shown by the difficulties encountered in performing quick, alternating movements in pronation–supination or flexion–extension [95]. PT programs must also include passive stretching of antagonist muscles and strengthening of agonist muscles [95]. Some exercises for active mobilization in axial rotation should be implemented to fight stiffness, which affects the trunk. Tai Chi exercises can also help to reduce balance disorders [78].

Transfers

As the disease progresses, complex motor sequences, such as transfers, may no longer be performed automatically [42]. Transfers that are particularly problematic include rising from, and sitting down onto a chair, getting in or out of bed, and turning over in bed [96]. A common problem during sit-to-stand transfers is that PD patients fail to lean forward far enough when standing up, thus falling back into the chair [41]. Cognitive cues would act as a potential facilitator of transfers. Motor strategies are designed to keep the gestures simple and easy, such as performing varied and repeated exercises dedicated to a precise daily activity to optimize training and facilitate transfers in the patient's daily life. Cued training could improve motor control during daily activities, such as the sit-to-stand task and rising from the bed in people with PD (Figs. 2.3 and 2.4). For example, sit-to-stand can be divided into four phases: "open legs," "move forward," "move upward," and "stand up."

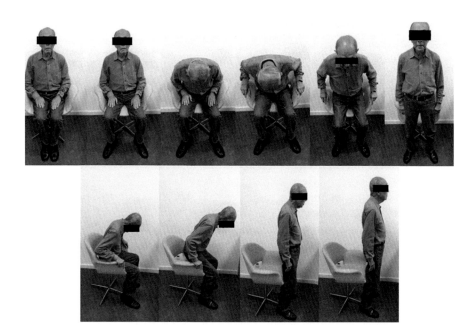

Fig. 2.3 Rising from the chair

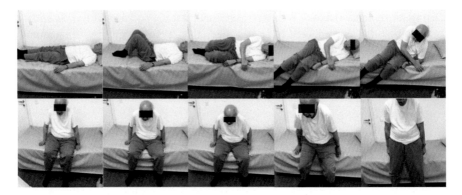

Fig. 2.4 Getting out of the bed

Manual Activities

Manual activities may become difficult to perform because of the complex motor sequences required. The coordination, efficiency, and speed of reach and dexterity of movements are often diminished; therefore, therapies may be directed at addressing loss of mobility, difficulties in reaching, grasping, and manipulating objects. and self-care activities such as eating and dressing. Nonstandardized techniques, commonly observational analysis or nonstandardized timed tasks, were most often used to assess impairments and activity limitations. There are limited formal clinical guidelines for treating and evaluating impairment of manual activities in PD patients.

Exercise

Studies on physical exercises with PD animal models have shown many plastic processes involved with neuroprotection mechanisms, such as angiogenesis improvement [97], increased anti-inflammatory responses [98], decreased inflammatory responses [99], and improvement of mitochondrial functions [100]. The neuroprotective effect of exercises in PD was also reported in rats trained on a treadmill [99–101].

It is possible that the main factors related to the neuroprotective effect of the physical exercise are neurotrophic factors such as the brain-derived neurotrophic factor (BDNF). These factors are essential to cellular differentiation, neuronal survival, migration, dendritic arborization, synaptogenesis, and synaptic plasticity [102]. BDNF expression is decreased in PD animal models [99–101] and in PD postmortem brains [103]. On the other hand, physical exercise is able to recover BDNF levels both in animal models [99–101, 104] and in patients with PD [105].

According to Petzinger et al. [106], exercise is beneficial for PD rehabilitation because it incorporates many aspects of practice important for goal-directed motor skill learning. These elements include repetition, intensity, and challenge, which together with skill training lead to improvement in motor performance.

Although there is a wide spectrum of exercise modalities, most of the studies share common elements, including *goal-based practice* for the acquisition of a skill, and *reinforcement* (learning through feedback). The feedback in turn serves to challenge patients beyond self-selected levels of perceived capability, maintaining motivation, and facilitating the engagement of individuals to become cognitively aware of movements that were previously automatic and unconscious [106].

Aerobic training is encouraged and all patients should exercise in their best medicated state. Shu et al. [107] conducted a meta-analysis study to evaluate the effectiveness of aerobic exercise for PD and suggested that aerobic exercise (including treadmill training, dancing, walking, and Tai Chi) might significantly improve motor action, balance, and gait, including gait velocity, stride/step length, and walking ability.

In relation to resistance training, a recent systematic review suggested that resistance training might have a positive effect on both muscle strength outcomes and functional outcomes. Resistance training was shown to increase fat-free mass, muscle strength, and improve mobility and performance in PD patients [108].

Most of the research target the motor symptoms of PD, but Reynolds et al. [109] reviewed the literature searching for the efficacy of aerobic and strengthening exercise interventions relative to mood, cognition, and sleep. The author concluded that aerobic and strengthening exercises offer especially promising treatment strategies for alleviating nonmotor symptoms of PD.

Despite a large number of studies demonstrating that exercise improves motor performance in PD, there is no consensus on which frequency and duration of treatment, number of repetitions, and difficulty/complexity of exercises should be endorsed [45]. Most of the studies adopt a global treatment program of 6–8 h distributed over 6–12 weeks, with 1–1.5 h of training per week. It has been suggested that intensive, specific exercise might improve rehabilitation outcomes for PD patients. To be considered an intensive program the exercise should be practiced 2–3 h/week for 6–14 weeks, totaling 12–42 h of treatment [110].

Based on the guideline of the American College of Sports Medicine (ACSM) van der Kolk and King [43] suggest the following exercises for PD: the program should include aerobic, strengthening, flexibility, and balance training. Aerobic training should be done 5 days/week for 30 min of moderate intensity or 3 days/week for 20 min at vigorous intensity. Strengthening should be performed 2 days/week, 8–10 exercises involving major muscle groups and 2 sets of 10–15 repetitions. Flexibility exercises should be done for 10 min each time. Balance training should be introduced for those who are at risk for falls. However, many PD patients present postural instability precociously; thus, balance exercise should be applied in accordance with patients' needs.

Other Interventions

Dance

Similarly, dance is receiving attention as an interesting exercise strategy for PD because it naturally combines cueing, spatial awareness, balance, strength and flexibility, and physical activity (or even aerobic exercise if sufficiently intense).

Dance can serve as an adjunct to traditional treatments to improve gait, balance, and QoL in people with PD [111]. Tango dance, specifically, has been shown in several studies to improve a multitude of motor and nonmotor features in people with PD [112–114], but other types of dance have been evaluated as well. A Cochrane review [115] included two dance studies in a large review of the effectiveness of PT interventions compared with no intervention in patients with PD. Their results suggested that dance might improve UPDRS motor scores (−8.48, CI −12.76 to −4.19), FOG (2.21, CI −4.63 to 0.22), and the 6-min walk test (6MWT; 38.94, −3.18 to 81.06) compared with no intervention. Through meta-analysis they indirectly compared dance randomized clinical trials (RCTs) with other PT intervention RCTs and concluded that there were no differences in the effectiveness of the PT interventions.

The Use of Virtual Reality as a Strategy for Physical Therapy in PD

Virtual reality (VR) is defined as a computerized simulation that allows users to interact with images and virtual objects that appear in the virtual environment in real time through multiple sensory modalities [116].

The application of VR to rehabilitation is based on the interaction of the person within a virtual environment, with the aim of promoting motor learning through enhanced perceptions (visual, auditory, and haptic inputs). In addition, such technology can be incorporated into games consoles offering a low-cost, user-friendly, and home-applicable device to promote physical activity.

Although the studies have small samples of patients and lack standardization of tools, systems, and methods, VR has shown promising results and its application in the rehabilitation of PD is growing. Investigation into how this instrument may optimally be adjusted to the specific needs of PD patients is required [117, 118].

Virtual reality training has many advantages compared with standard physical rehabilitation interventions. It offers augmented feedback about performance, enables individualized practice, and stimulates both motor and cognitive functions simultaneously. Nonetheless, there are many challenging issues to be overcome. It is mandatory to better define suitable patients and establish the minimum cognitive and motor function for VR intervention, design better well-powered clinical trials, develop good assessment tools to measure the outcomes, and carry out long-term studies to measure learning and retention (Table 2.1).

Future Directions

Physical therapy has been indicated as adjuvant to pharmacological and surgical treatments in PD. It should be recommended as early as possible to maximize functional abilities, to improve QoL, and to minimize secondary complications. However, past meta-analysis studies showed insufficient evidence to support or refute the efficacy of PT. In the last decade, both the number and quality of RCTs have increased substantially and different interventions, such as exercise, are now accepted and regarded as basic elements of any rehabilitation program. Many questions remain unanswered, but large and well-designed ongoing trials are promising to increase the current levels of evidence that support the use of PT strategies, e.g., to prevent falls or to improve physical capacity in PD patients.

Table 2.1 Virtual reality in Parkinson's disease (PD)

Reference	Intervention or assessment	Aim of the intervention
Souza et al. [55]	Intervention	Combined visual and auditory cues on walking after deep brain stimulation
Yang et al. [186]	Intervention	To improve gait, balance, posture, and freezing
Cipresso et al. [187]	Assessment	Virtual multiple errands test (VMET) to evaluate executive function
Su et al. [188]	Assessment	Postural instability
Shine et al. [189]	Assessment	Freezing of gait
Griffin et al. [190]	Intervention	Use of virtual visual cues on walking
Mirelman et al. [118]	Intervention	Motor–cognitive training and obstacle negotiation
Yen et al. [191]	Intervention	Training balance in a single- or dual-task condition
Albani et al. [192]	Intervention	To improve executive function with virtual reality
Davidsdottir et al. [193]	Assessment	Visual processing during gait
Albani et al. [194]	Intervention	To improve daily activities in the virtual reality home environment

Speech Therapy in Parkinson's Disease

Introduction

Motor and nonmotor deficits affect the abilities of communication and swallowing and can have a devastating impact on the QoL of patients with PD.

These impairments pose management challenges to physicians and speech therapists. Rehabilitation plans should take an interdisciplinary approach and combine dopaminergic and nondopaminergic drug therapies with nonpharmacological interventions to manage patients.

Language–speech therapy, including targeted training with systematic, repeated, and controlled actions, can help to overcome the neurochemical loss and reduce specific symptoms of the disease.

Organic Neurological Dysphonia

The voice is affected earlier than other subsystems of verbal communication and impairments can be identified before the diagnosis of PD. Around 70–80 % of individuals with PD have dysphonia [119]. Changes in voice characteristics vary as they may have variable degrees of magnitude.

Dysphonia is analyzed by auditory–perceptual evaluation, automatic computerized acoustic (spectral and cepstral modeling, sound pressure level, fundamental frequency, jitter, shimmer, amplitude perturbation quotient, pitch perturbation quotient, noise content measures, prosodic features, nonlinear behavior, stability, periodicity features), laryngostroboscopic, aerodynamics, and subjective self-rating questionnaire, which can add additional information necessary for biological and physiological data associated with voice disorders.

Surgical and pharmacological treatments that have a significant impact on motor symptoms have shown limited effectiveness on communication skills for most PD patients [120].

Speech–language therapy rehabilitation is aimed at recovering the voice through exercises, techniques, and methods. The Lee Silverman Voice Treatment (LSVT or LSVT LOUD) improves vocal intensity and phonation [121, 122].

Hypokinetic Dysarthria

Dysarthria is seen in as many as 90 % of individuals with PD [123]. These patients experience changes in speech and voice and when verbal communication skills deteriorate, speech becomes unintelligible. This manifestation is caused by muscle control and sensory integration dysfunction and can affect respiration, phonation, resonance, articulation, and prosody.

Voice disorders tend to increase as the disease progresses, whereas speech disorders are associated with advanced stages of PD [124], bradykinesia, and axial motor deficits [125]. The assessments of dysarthria and dysphonia are similar and it is essential to evaluate the patient with PD to differentiate the type of the deficits.

Drug and neurosurgical treatment are insufficient and have variable results for dysarthria in PD [126]. The specific effects of DBS and repetitive transcranial magnetic stimulation and related mechanisms remain unknown.

When initiated, the speech–language therapy rehabilitation program consists of an integrated approach, including guidance, psychodynamic interventions, and training.

The multiple barriers of access to this intensive treatment faced by patients with PD include their own physical limitations, long distances to the treatment center, lack of transportation services, and requiring a travel companion to get to the rehabilitation center [127]. To overcome these barriers, the LSVT was tested for remote delivery. The results were encouraging, and the improvements obtained were similar to those with on-site rehabilitation [128].

Telerehabilitation should be weighed up carefully. Factors such as aging, digital inclusion, and lifestyle in addition to cultural, social, and economic characteristics, need to be taken into account, as patients may refuse this form of treatment [129]. The clinical practice guidelines for synchronous telerehabilitation require users to comply with standards of storage, handling, and transmission of data to ensure patient protection, privacy, and confidentiality (Table 2.2).

Table 2.2 Aspects of dysphonia and dysarthria

Features	Changes	Signs	Impact	Treatment
Voice quality	Breathiness, tremor, harshness	Irregular vibration of vocal folds; transglottic air escape noise not set to sound phonation	Noise phonation, breathy voice	Lee Silverman Voice Treatment, pitch limiting voice treatment (PLVT)
Voice intensity	Hypophonia	Vocal fold bowing, incomplete vocal fold closure	Reduced loudness	Lee Silverman Voice Treatment
Monopitch	Dysprosody	Rigidity of vocal folds	Monotone speech	Lee Silverman Voice Treatment, PLVT
Monoloudness	Dysprosody	Rigidity of vocal folds	Monotone speech	Lee Silverman Voice Treatment, PLVT
Articulation	Imprecision of pronunciation	Akinesia, bradykinesia, rigidity	Impaired speech intelligibility	Lee Silverman Voice Treatment, articulatory training
Reduced speed	Slow speech	Bradykinesia	Monotone speech	Metronome, delayed auditory feedback, medication
Increased speed	Rapid speech	Rigidity	Impaired speech intelligibility	Metronome, delayed auditory feedback, medication
Palilalia	Dysfluency	Bradykinesia, tremor	Interruptions, pauses, hesitations, repetitions	Medication

Studies have shown that the LSVT produces functional benefits in various sub-systems of verbal communication, such as voice quality, prosody, articulation, and speech intelligibility, and it is thus a useful therapeutic option [130]. The levels of evidence of treatment for PD with LSVT are as follows: European Federation of Neurological Societies and Movement Disorder Society (EFNS/MDS): class B—level II [131]; National Institute for Health and Clinical Excellence (NICE): class B—level II [132]; Guidelines for Speech–Language Therapy in Parkinson's Disease (Concept Translation Parkinsonnet): class A—level I [133].

Language Dysfunction

It is estimated that 50–60 % of PD patients experience impaired language under-standing and expression (cognitive-linguistic disturbances). These manifestations are related to language processing, cognitive or neuropsychological deficits and cognitive-neuropsychological impairments.

Therefore, effects of bradyphrenia, deficits in verbal working memory, prob-lems with set-shifting, poor attention and distractibility, dual-task processing factors, executive dysfunction, among others, are associated with language dif-ficulties [134].

Although voice and speech changes have been widely investigated and rehabili-tation approaches are recognized and extensively studied, so far there is no specific treatment designed for language improvement in PD. Systematic studies are neces-sary to better understand and manage language disorders in PD. This is a wide-open area of investigation.

Other Verbal and Nonverbal Communication Disorders

Parkinson's disease also involves nonverbal language impairment. This manifesta-tion is associated with dysphonia or dysarthria and further undermines communica-tion in social, professional, and family environments.

Written communication is greatly affected by dysgraphia, which is characterized by micrography, and prevents partial or total reading of the written content pro-duced. In this sense, writing can be optimized by typing the content using a com-puter, smartphone or tablet or any other similar device. However, motor deficits in hands and fingers hinder these tasks.

Conversation involves a variety of non-verbal messages such as body postures and movements, arm and hand gestures, smiles, glances, and facial expressions to signal the individual's intention to start a conversation and take his or her turn.

Facial expressions help to convey the intent of the speech. Hypomimia is a common feature in PD that makes it difficult for listeners to understand patients with PD and to perceive their general and affective states [135, 136]. The LSVT may also help to improve these patients' facial expressions and communication (Table 2.3).

Table 2.3 Other aspects of communication

Features	Changes	Signs	Impact	Treatment
Dysgraphia	Micrography	Bradykinesia, akinesia, rigidity	Handwriting impairment	Manual training, medication
Hypomimia	Masked facies	Bradykinesia, akinesia, rigidity	Inefficient facial expression	LSVT, medication

Oropharyngeal Dysphagia

Dysphagia is very common in PD. It affects up to 80 % of individuals in the early stages and as many as 95 % in the advanced stages of the disease because of motor and nonmotor deficits [137]. Difficulty swallowing is most frequently associated with the oral and pharyngeal phases, resulting in inefficient bolus formation, delayed swallowing reflex, slowed pharyngeal transit time, and repetitive swallowing to push food toward the esophagus and clear the glottic region [138].

Treatment standards of dysphagia in patients with PD were elaborate according to the stages of swallowing: (1) oral (voluntary): repetitive pump movements of the tongue, oral residue, premature spillage, piecemeal deglutition; (2) pharyngeal (involuntary): residue in valleculae, pyriform sinuses, aspiration, somatosensory deficits, reduced rate of spontaneous swallows; (3) esophageal (involuntary): hypomotility, spasms, and multiple contractions [139].

Clinical observation has revealed that patients with PD also have difficulty in other phases of swallowing. During the anticipatory phase, patients lose the ability to choose the right foods, control the amount of food and set the pace of eating. Many patients tend to choose inadequately dry or hard solid foods and quickly put an excessive amount of food into their mouth. During the oral preparatory phase, they have difficulty holding cups and using cutlery to bring food to their mouth and/or lack the strength to close their lips and teeth and hold food inside their mouth.

Dysphagia can produce two different sets of complications, with an impact on the overall health of patients: (a) malnutrition and/or dehydration due to reduced effectiveness of swallowing; and (b) choking and tracheobronchial aspiration caused by impaired safety of swallowing, which result in respiratory infections and aspiration pneumonia.

Fiber-optic endoscopic evaluation of swallowing and videofluoroscopy swallowing studies are considered the gold standard for evaluation of oropharyngeal dysphagia [140], but should be combined with rigorous speech therapy analysis to guide the management of rehabilitation.

Dysphagia may be treated by rehabilitation, surgical or pharmacological methods or with other approaches (dental implants, overdentures, percutaneous injection of botulinum toxin).

Surgery is rarely indicated for patients with swallowing disorders, although in patients with severe disorders, bypassing the oral cavity and pharynx in their entirety and providing enteral nutrition may be necessary. Options include percutaneous endoscopic gastrostomy and intermittent oro-esophageal catheterization [141].

Some studies have demonstrated that DBS did not show clinically significant improvement or decline in swallowing. Evidence shows that subthalamic nucleus (STN) stimulation appears to cause more impairment than globus pallidus internus (GPi) stimulation [142].

As for drug treatment, although few studies have shown improved swallowing after ingestion of levodopa, several studies have reported improved dysphagia with dopaminergic treatment in only a small proportion of patients. In these cases, behavioral therapy should be considered [143].

Speech–language therapy rehabilitation is key for improving dysphagia and includes both *compensatory* strategies and *rehabilitation* techniques [144]. The compensatory intervention is produced by chin-tuck, bolus consistency, effortful swallow frequency, and bolus effects. Rehabilitation consists of tongue-strengthening, tongue control, tongue holder, Shaker technique, and vocal exercises.

Learned compensatory maneuvers as part of the behavioral intervention for dysphagia including changing the diet, the way food is eaten, head posture, and adjusting the swallowing mechanism.

Changes in diet aim to create different sensory stimulation, for example, by changing volume, texture, and consistency of the food. Changes in head posture such as rotating or tilting it backward or forward can help move and increase the flow of the bolus. As for the swallowing mechanism, it can be improved with several maneuvers, including the Shaker maneuver, supraglottic swallow, super supraglottic swallow, the Masako maneuver, and the Mendelsohn maneuver to adjust muscle strength, range of motion, and coordination between swallowing and breathing

Sialorrhea

As there are no established diagnostic criteria for sialorrhea, prevalence estimates of drooling and sialorrhea in patients with PD vary from 10 to 84 % [145]. These manifestations are more common during the *off* periods, probably because of increased production or insufficient clearance of saliva [146].

Oropharyngeal dysphagia and lack of upper esophageal motility are the main factors contributing to drooling and sialorrhea [147]. Hypomimia, unintentional opening of the mouth, and bent posture of the head may be secondary causes [148].

The evaluation of drooling in PD includes objective measures (volume and salivary flow) and subjective (Unified Parkinson's Disease Rating Scale part II, Drooling Severity and Frequency Scale, Drooling Rating Scale, and Sialorrhea Clinical Scale for PD). The Movement Disorders Society recommends the use of all subjective measures.

Treatment should begin by discontinuing, if possible, all medications that exacerbate drooling and sialorrhea, such as cholinesterase inhibitors, clozapine or quetiapine. The goal is to improve motor deficit symptoms using dopaminergic medications or DBS. However, response to treatment is usually partial and requires specific adjuvant therapy. Pharmacological and nonpharmacological treatments are recommended. Anticholinergics, adrenergic receptor antagonists, and botulinum neurotoxin of serotypes A and B, have been utilized.

Table 2.4 Dysphagia, drooling and sialorrhea

Features	Changes	Signs	Impact	Treatment
Dysphagia	Coughing, gagging, difficulty swallowing foods and drugs	Bradykinesia, rigidity, akinesia, incomplete cricopharyngeal relaxation, reduced cricopharyngeal opening, delayed initiation of the swallowing reflex	Aspiration, pneumonia, malnutrition, death	LSVT, swallowing training, medication
Drooling and sialorrhea	Impairment in speech and feeding, saliva escape through the mouth	Lingual bradykinesia, dysphagia, changes in upper esophageal motility, hypomimia, head posture	Pneumonia aspiration saliva, perioral dermatitis, bad breath	Swallowing training, medication

Speech–language therapy rehabilitation may improve patients' ability to retain saliva within the mouth, but further studies are needed to investigate its effectiveness (Table 2.4).

Future Directions

Communication and swallowing disorders affect most patients with PD and have an adverse impact on their functioning. Because evidence shows that patients with these presentations respond inconsistently and weakly to pharmacological or neurosurgical treatment alone, language–speech rehabilitation should be recommended, as studies suggest significant improvement of these functions after therapy.

So far, there is /little evidence supporting the effectiveness of currently used interventions and they need further validation. Future studies involving other treatment research areas may help to clarify the neural basis of communication and swallowing disorders in PD and drive the development and improvement of treatment approaches. Furthermore, progress in rehabilitation is achieved with national and international collaborative work and sharing of research data.

Occupational Therapy Intervention in Patients with Parkinson's Disease

Introduction

The progress of PD leads to loss of the abilities to perform ADLs and subsequently poor functional status and worse QoL. The impairments become gradually evident, making it essential for the patient and the caregiver to be oriented and trained to avoid any secondary damage [149]. During the course of the disease, the patient with PD requires the help of allied health professionals, such as the occupational therapist.

Occupational therapy (OT) intervention can be conducted at the patient's home or in the rehabilitation center (as an outpatient). There is no consensus on which place is more effective for the rehabilitation process [150, 151]. However, it is agreed that the therapist should target the activities and exercises that are significant for the patient. The family/caregiver must understand the patient's deficits and goals so that they may motivate the patients to practice the occupational therapist's exercises at home and improve their QoL.

Patients may take a long time to perform ADLs, not only because of the motor impairment (such a, freezing, tremor, and bradykinesia), but also because of the cognitive deficits. These deficits may also interfere with the performance of more complex tasks, such as paying the bills and taking medication [152]. For this reason, OT interventions should be tailored to address the multiple physical and psychosocial difficulties that PD patients may face. Simplifying the activity or breaking down complex tasks into simple steps may be necessary in some cases. Moreover, patients may require some tips/cues, assistance or supervision to complete ADLs [153].

Each patient requires different strategies of intervention, for motor impairments, such as balance, freezing, and coordination. A more accessible environment can be created to avoid falls and secondary consequences (e.g., fractures) [152]. At home, adaptations (such as bars, ramps, raised toilet seats, and stair lifts) should be evaluated by the therapist and the adjustments recommended to the patients. Sometimes, only the simplest orientations (such as removing mats and furniture) can be helpful in avoiding falls. Safety and awareness of the deficits are essential for the patients to improve functional status and QoL.

As discussed, patients with PD have multiple aspects to be considered and evaluated at the initial assessment and during different phases of the disease. All the difficulties and abilities of the patients with PD have to be considered to provide an adequate rehabilitation program. It is also important that frequent reassessments are made to change the treatment goals accordingly [154].

Although there is a lack of studies measuring OT intervention in PD, and consequently evidence of its effectiveness in the rehabilitation process is limited [149, 150, 155–157], meta-analysis studies have been performed with the aim of drawing out more data about OT assessment and treatment [153, 158, 159]. Most of the studies approach the following aspects that should be emphasized when evaluating patients with PD: (1) motor aspects, (2) cognitive deficits, (3) ADLs and Instrumental Activities of Daily Living (IADL), (4) home environment, and (5) family/caregiver support. In the following section these topics are addressed.

Motor Aspects

The majority of patients with PD are sedentary and during the course of the disease, they will experience loss of motor function and balance and may have trouble initiating a motor action, such as walking and transfers (e.g., bed to chair). Exercises and activities to promote stretching, strengthening, and balance are important to retard the decaying of these functions [154]. Physical activities are also important for the patient's QoL and improvement of functional status [160], which in turn prevents comorbidities and avoids hospitalization [161, 162].

At the initial assessment, upper limb function should be evaluated. Proud et al. [163] investigated the frequency of physiotherapy and OT assessment of the upper limb in people with PD. The results showed that only 54 % of respondents regularly assessed upper limb function. Therefore, effort should be made to increase clinicians' knowledge of appropriate outcome measures for quantifying upper limb impairments and activity limitations that may be addressed in this population [164].

Practice and training different postures to perform the daily routine tasks are recommended, such as a sitting position for showering/bathing or putting clothes in the *on/off* period. Assistive technology and utensils such as: eating and drinking tools, dressing tools, computer aids, cooking tools, and bathroom aids, among others, may help the patient with PD to be more independent [165].

There are few studies addressing splinting for patients with PD; however, its benefits for other neurological diseases are well known [166]. The splints can be used to prevent the stress of ligament, muscle, joint or correct deformity [166]. PD patients may experience stiffness of the hand, pain and loss of range of movement with the progression of the disease, but there is no specific splinting for each patient. The occupational therapist should evaluate the motor aspects and discuss the goals with the patient and family/caregiver, before recommending a splint.

During the progress of the PD, patients lose the walking ability for a short or long distance due to imbalance, rigidity, and freezing. These impairments can provoke falls and fatigue. For this reason, the occupational therapist should evaluate the patient's needs and discuss the prescription of a wheelchair and shower chair [167]. Patient and family may have concerns about using a wheelchair, but it is important to explain all the reasons for its indication, especially to prevent secondary problems caused by falls.

Cognitive Aspects

Mild cognitive impairment and dementia can develop during the progression of PD in approximately 30 % of the patients [168–170]. The most common cognitive impairments are memory, attention, visuospatial, and executive function [156, 168].

The Movement Disorders Society Parkinson Study Group Cognitive/Psychiatric Working Group recommends Montreal Cognitive Assessment [171] as a minimum cognitive screening measure in clinical trials of PD where cognitive performance is not the primary outcome [172]. Mini Mental State Examination [173] is another useful screening instrument for assessment of cognitive impairment in PD [174].

Patients may require some tips/cues or supervision to perform ADLs, such as remembering the timing of medications, appointments or even more complex tasks (paying the bills and simple meal preparation). People with PD may experience difficulties in performing dual tasks (e.g., walking and carrying a cup or walking and looking for a product on the supermarket shelf), owing to the motor aspects, but also because of divided attention [154, 175, 176].

Activities of Daily Living and Instrumental Activities of Daily Living

Activities of daily living are difficult for people with PD; there are many causes, including fatigue, slowness, fear/risk of falling, depression, and effects of medication [154, 177]. It is important to stimulate the patients to perform daily tasks and to maintain their own autonomy and independence.

Encouragement to have some leisure activities (social and cultural activities) is essential, not only for meeting friends and family, but also for having some time off from the weekly routine. Although there are few studies about the benefits of leisure and social activities for patients with PD, studies indicate that older people who participate in these activities present reduced cognitive decline [156, 178].

Patients should participate not only in their family's events, but also in religious groups, friends' groups, clubs, and volunteer work [178]. The therapist should also recommend that the patients participate in support groups for PD, outdoor activities (cinema, theater, and park), and practice arm/hand motor skills. Group activities are beneficial for patients to discuss experiences, difficulties, and abilities, and to cope with the disease [70, 179].

The suggested questionnaires for evaluating the ADLs and IADL in patients with Parkinson's are: the Canadian Occupational Performance Measure [180] and the Parkinson Self-Assessment Tool [181].

Home Environment

During the rehabilitation process it is important to evaluate the patient's home and work place to make it accessible, comfortable, safe, and functional. It is essential to discuss with the patient and family their needs for an adequate housing and environmental adaptation [151, 182].

Family/Caregiver Support

Family/caregivers should understand the patients' potential and limitations and the treatment process. Dependence and incapacity cause emotional problems for patients and consequently affect the family/caregiver, who should be encouraged to participate in a family support group. Studies demonstrate that QoL in patients with PD and their caregiving spouses is decreased. Multidisciplinary interventions aimed at improving PD patients' QoL may have more effective outcomes if education about coping skills targeted not only patients, but also family/caregivers [183–185]. The family/caregivers' burdens increase as the patients' limitations increase and there is a need for good wellbeing. It is important to take into consideration their issues of concern in relation to the patient and the disease (Table 2.5).

Table 2.5 Occupational therapy interventions in PD

Intervention	Suggested activities	Local	PD progression
Exercises to improve motor activities	Exercises to practice the movements and functions of the upper limb, such as reaching, gripping, grasping and manipulating the objects	Clinic and home	During the progression of PD, activities should change according to the patient's needs
Cognitive activities	Virtual games, attention games, outdoor activities, group activities, board games, tablet games	Clinic	As soon as the patient presents cognitive impairments
Practice and orientation for the ADL and IADL	Different posture to dress and bath Practice of transferences (bed–chair; chair–wheelchair) Practice of housekeeping and cooking Outdoor activities, such as grocery, bank and cultural activities Adaptation and devices to facilitate the daily activities	The best place for this intervention is in the patient's environment; however, it can be done at the clinic	As soon as the patient presents first symptoms with an impact on their functional status
Assessment of home environment	When patient presents the initial symptom of PD, the OT should investigate the patient's environment Recommendations for avoiding falls should be addressed Equipment (e.g., raised toilet seat and bars) and refurbishment (e.g., ramp, lift or even more spacious bedroom and bathroom) Simple adaptations, such as: removal of mats; moving the patient's bedroom to the living room; removal of the door frame, installation of bars, and use of a chair to have a shower (or even a strip wash)	Home and Workstation	At the initial assessment and according to the progression of the disease
Family and caregiver support	Posture to assist the patient and avoid pain Organize the patient's and caregiver's routine Family support groups Time to relax and run errands Caregiver support group to share experiences	Clinic or at home	During the progression of the disease

All the activities and exercises should be practiced (at least for the first time) with the OT, but the caregiver should also practice with the patient at home to improve the functional status

Future Directions

People with PD require professional health care during the whole course of the disease; however, there is a lack of evidence for the effectiveness of OT intervention. A few of the reasons: there are not enough randomized clinical trials, not enough financial support to conduct large trials, and insufficient health professionals specialized in PD to conduct research. More multicenter clinical trials to evaluate all the aspects that involve OT interventions in patients with PD should be encouraged in the future.

References

1. Schrag A. Epidemiology of movement disorders. In: Jankovic J, Tolosa E, editors. Parkinson's disease and movement disorders. Baltimore: Lippincott; 2007. p. 50–2.
2. Bach JP, Ziegler U, Deuschl G, Dodel R, Doblhammer-Reiter G. Projected numbers of people with movement disorders in the years 2030 and 2050. Mov Disord. 2011;26:2286–90.
3. Gibb WRG, Lees AJ. The relevance of the Lewy body to the pathogenesis of idiopathic Parkinson's disease. J Neurol Neurosurg Psychiatry. 1988;51:745–52.
4. Braak H, Ghebremedhin E, Rüb U, Bratzke H, Del Tredici K. Stages in the development of Parkinson's disease-related pathology. Cell Tissue Res. 2004;318:121–34.
5. Van Maele-Fabry G, Hoet P, Vilain F, Lison D. Occupational exposure to pesticides and Parkinson's disease: a systematic review and meta-analysis of cohort studies. Environ Int. 2012;46:30–43.
6. Kandinov B, Giladi N, Korczyn AD. The effect of cigarette smoking, tea, and coffee consumption on the progression of Parkinson's disease. Parkinsonism Relat Disord. 2007;13:243–5.
7. Quik M, Perez XA, Bordia T. Nicotine as a potential neuroprotective agent for Parkinson's disease. Mov Disord. 2012;27:947–57.
8. Sääksjärvi K, Knekt P, Rissanen H, Laaksonen MA, Reunanen A, Männistö S. Prospective study of coffee consumption and risk of Parkinson's disease. Eur J Clin Nutr. 2008;62:908–15.
9. Derkinderen P, Shannon KM, Brundin P. Gut feelings about smoking and coffee in Parkinson's disease. Mov Disord. 2014;29:976–9.
10. Polymeropoulos MH, Lavedan C, Leroy E, Ide SE, Dehejia A, Dutra A, et al. Mutation in the alpha-synuclein gene identified in families with Parkinson's disease. Science. 1997;276:2045–7.
11. de Lau LM, Breteler MM. Epidemiology of Parkinson's disease. Lancet Neurol. 2006;5:525–35.
12. Fearnley JM, Lees AJ. Ageing and Parkinson's disease: substantia nigra regional selectivity. Brain. 1991;114:2283–301.
13. Ma SY, Röytt M, Collan Y, Rinne JO. Unbiased morphometrical measurements show loss of pigmented nigral neurones with ageing. Neuropathol Appl Neurobiol. 1999;25:394–9.
14. Pakkenberg B, Møller A, Gundersen HJ, Mouritzen Dam A, Pakkenberg H. The absolute number of nerve cells in substantia nigra in normal subjects and in patients with Parkinson's disease estimated with an unbiased stereological method. J Neurol Neurosurg Psychiatry. 1991;54:31.
15. Lashuel HA, Overk CR, Oueslati A, Masliah E. The many faces of α-synuclein: from structure and toxicity to therapeutic target. Nat Rev Neurosci. 2013;14:38–48.
16. Chu Y, Kordower JH. Lewy body pathology in fetal grafts. Ann N Y Acad Sci. 2010;1184:55–67.
17. Winklhofer K, Haass C. Mitochondrial dysfunction in Parkinson's disease. Biochim Biophys Acta. 2010;1802:29–44.

18. Kannarkat GT, Boss JM, Tansey MG. The role of innate and adaptive immunity in Parkinson's disease. J Parkinsons Dis. 2013;3:493–514.
19. Appel SH. Inflammation in Parkinson's disease: cause or consequence? Mov Disord. 2012;27:1075–7.
20. Speciali DS, Corrêa JC, Luna NM, Brant R, Greve JM, de Godoy W, et al. Validation of GDI, GPS and GVS for use in Parkinson's disease through evaluation of effects of subthalamic deep brain stimulation and levodopa. Gait Posture. 2014;39:1142–5.
21. Hughes AJ, Ben-Shlomo Y, Daniel SE, Lees AJ. What features improve the accuracy of clinical diagnosis in Parkinson's disease: a clinicopathologic study. Neurology. 1992;42:1142–6.
22. Hughes AJ, Daniel SE, Kilford L, Lees AJ. Accuracy of clinical diagnosis of idiopathic Parkinson's disease: a clinico-pathological study of 100 cases. J Neurol Neurosurg Psychiatry. 1992;55:181–4.
23. Josephs KA, Dickson DW. Diagnostic accuracy of progressive supranuclear palsy in the society for progressive supranuclear palsy brain bank. Mov Disord. 2003;18:1018–26.
24. Gilman S, Wenning GK, Low PA, Brooks DJ, Mathias CJ, Trojanowski JQ, et al. Second consensus statement on the diagnosis of multiple system atrophy. Neurology. 2008;71:670–6.
25. Felicio AC, Godeiro-Junior C, Shih MC, Borges V, Silva SM, Aguiar Pde C, et al. Evaluation of patients with clinically unclear parkinsonian syndromes submitted to brain SPECT imaging using the technetium-99m labeled tracer TRODAT-1. J Neurol Sci. 2010;291:64–8.
26. Bor-Seng-Shu E, Fonoff ET, Barbosa ER, Teixeira MJ. Substantia nigra hyperechogenicity in Parkinson's disease. Acta Neurochir (Wien). 2010;152:2085–7.
27. Silveira-Moriyama L, Carvalho Mde J, Katzenschlager R, Petrie A, Ranvaud R, Barbosa ER, et al. The use of smell tests in the diagnosis of PD in Brazil. Mov Disord. 2008;23:2328–34.
28. Cochrane CJ, Ebmeier KP. Diffusion tensor imaging in parkinsonian syndromes. A systematic review and meta-analysis. Neurology. 2013;80:857–64.
29. Vaillancourt DE, Spraker MB, Prodoehl J, Abraham I, Corcos DM, Zhou XJ, et al. High-resolution diffusion tensor imaging in the substantia nigra of de novo Parkinson disease. Neurology. 2009;72:378–84.
30. Schwarz ST, Abaei M, Gontu V, Morgan PS, Bajaj N, Auer DP. Diffusion tensor imaging of nigral degeneration in Parkinson's disease: a region-of-interest and voxel-based study at 3T and systematic review with meta-analysis. NeuroImage. 2013;3:481–8.
31. Al-Bachari S, Parkes LM, Vidyasagar R, Hnaby MF, Tharaken V, Leroi I, et al. Arterial spin labelling reveals prolonged arterial arrival time in idiopathic Parkinson's disease. NeuroImage. 2014;6:1–8.
32. Olanow CW, Stern MB, Sethi K. The scientific and clinical basis for the treatment of Parkinson disease. Neurology. 2009;72 Suppl 4:S1–136.
33. Rajput AH. Levodopa prolongs life expectancy and is non-toxic to substantia nigra. Parkinsonism Relat Disord. 2001;8:95–100.
34. Parkinson Study Group. Pramipexole vs levodopa as initial treatment for Parkinson disease: a randomized controlled trial. Parkinson Study group. JAMA. 2000;284:1931–8.
35. Witjas T, Kaphan E, Azulay JP, Blin O, Ceccaldi M, Pouget J, et al. Nonmotor fluctuations in Parkinson's disease: frequent and disabling. Neurology. 2002;59:408–13.
36. Olanow CW, Rascol O, Hauser R, et al. A double-blind, delayed-start trial of rasagiline in Parkinson's disease. N Engl J Med. 2009;361:1268–78.
37. Rascol O, Brooks DJ, Melamed E, Oertel W, Poewe W, Stocchi F, et al. Rasagiline as an adjunct to levodopa in patients with Parkinson's disease and motor fluctuations (LARGO, lasting effect in adjunct therapy with rasagiline given once daily, study): a randomised, double-blind, parallel-group trial. Lancet. 2005;365:947–54.
38. Schüepbach WM, Knudsen K, Volkmann J, Krack P, Timmermann L, Hälbig TD, et al. EARLYSTIM Study Group. Neurostimulation for Parkinson's disease with early motor complications. N Engl J Med. 2013;368:610–22.
39. DeLong MR, Huang KT, Gallis J, Lokhnygina Y, Parente B, Hickey P, et al. Effect of advancing age on outcomes of deep brain stimulation for Parkinson disease. JAMA Neurol. 2014;71:1290–5.

40. Factor SA, Bennett A, Hohler AD, Wang D, Miyasaki JM. Quality improvement in neurology: Parkinson disease update quality measurement set: executive summary. Neurology. 2016;86(24):2278–83. doi:10.1212/WNL.0000000000002670.
41. Keus SHJ, Bloem BR, Hendriks EJ, Bredero-Cohen AB, Munneke M. Practice Recommendations Development Group. Evidence-based analysis of physical therapy in Parkinson's disease with recommendations for practice and research. Mov Disord. 2007;22:451–60.
42. Keus SHJ, Munneke M, Graziano M, Paltamaa J, Pelosin E, Domingos J, et al. European Physiotherapy Guideline for Parkinson's disease. 2014; KNGF/ParkinsonNet.
43. Van der Kolk NM, King LA. Effects of exercise on mobility in people with Parkinson's disease. Mov Disord. 2013;15(28):1587–96.
44. Debaere F, Wenderoth N, Sunaert S, Van Hecke P, Swinnen SP. Internal vs external generation of movements: differential neural pathways involved in bimanual coordination performed in the presence or absence of augmented visual feedback. Neuroimage. 2003;19:764–76.
45. Goodwin VA, Richards SH, Taylor RS, Taylor AH, Campbell JL. The effectiveness of exercise interventions for people with Parkinson's disease: a systematic review and meta-analysis. Mov Disord. 2008;15(23):631–40.
46. Soh SE, Morris ME, McGinley JL. Determinants of health-related quality of life in Parkinson's disease: a systematic review. Parkinsonism Relat Disord. 2011;8:1–9.
47. Maetzler W, Nieuwhof F, Hasmann SE, Bloem BR. Emerging therapies for gait disability and balance impairment: promises and pitfalls. Mov Disord. 2013;28:1576–86.
48. Lim I, Van Wegen E, De Goede C, Deutekom M, Niewboer A, Willems A, et al. Effects of external rhythmical cueing on gait in patients with Parkinson's disease: a systematic review. Clin Rehabil. 2005;19:695–713.
49. Nieuwboer A. Cueing for freezing of gait in patients with Parkinson's disease: a rehabilitation perspective. Mov Disord. 2008;23:475–81.
50. Rochester L, Burn DJ, Woods G, Godwin J, Nieuwboer A. Does auditory rhythmical cueing improve gait in people with Parkinson's disease and cognitive impairment? A feasibility study. Mov Disord. 2009;24:839–45.
51. Donovan S, Lim C, Diaz N, Browner N, Rose P, Sudarsky LR. Laserlight cues for gait freezing in Parkinson's disease: an open-label study. Parkinsonism Relat Disord. 2011;17:240–5.
52. Bunting-Perry L, Spindler M, Robinson K, Noorigian MJ, Cianci HJ, Duda JE. Laser light visual cueing for freezing of gait in Parkinson disease: a pilot study with male participants. J Rehabil Res Dev. 2013;50:223–30.
53. Ferrarin M, Brambilla M, Garavello L, Di Candia A, Pedotti A, Rabuffetti M. Microprocessor-controlled optical stimulating device to improve the gait of patients with Parkinson's disease. Med Biol Eng Comput. 2004;42:328–32.
54. Lopez-Contreras WO, Higuera CA, Fonoff ET, Souza CO, Albicker U, Martinez JA. Listenmee and Listenmee smartphone application: synchronizing walking to rhythmic auditory cues to improve gait in Parkinson's disease. Hum Mov Sci. 2014;37:147–56.
55. Souza CO, Voos MC, Chien HF, Brant R, Barbosa AF, Barbosa ER, et al. Combined auditory and visual cuing provided by eyeglasses influence gait performance in Parkinson disease patients submitted to DBS: a pilot study. Int Arch Med. 2015;8:132–8.
56. Amboni M, Barone P, Luppariello L, Lista I, Transfaglia R, Fasano A, et al. Gait patterns in parkinsonian patients with or without mild cognitive impairment. Mov Disord. 2012;27:1536–43.
57. Martin KL, Blizzard L, Wood AG, Srikanth V, Thomson R, Sanders LM, et al. Cognitive function, gait and gait variability in older people: a population-based study. J Gerontol A Biol Sci Med Sci. 2012;68:726–32.
58. Srygley JM, Mirelman A, Gilai N, Hausdorff JM. When does walking alter thinking? Age and task associated findings. Brain Res. 2009;1253:92–9.
59. Allcock LM, Rowan EN, Steen IN, Wesnes K, Kenny RA, Burn DJ. Impaired attention predicts falling in Parkinson's disease. Parkinsonism Relat Disord. 2009;15:110–15.

60. Bouquet CA, Bonnaud V, Gil R. Investigation of supervisory attentional system functions in patients with Parkinson's disease using the Hayling task. J Clin Exp Neuropsychol. 2003;25:751–60.
61. Rochester L, Hetherington V, Jones D, Nieuwboer A, Willems A, Kwakkel G, et al. Attending to the task: interference effects of functional tasks on walking in Parkinson's disease and the roles of cognition, depression, fatigue, and balance. Arch Phys Med Rehabil. 2004;85(10):1578–85.
62. Yogev G, Giladi N, Gruendlinger L, Baltadjieva R, Simon E, Hausdorff J. Executive function, mental loading and gait variability in Parkinson's disease. J Am Geriatr Soc. 2004;52 Suppl 3:S3.
63. Ebersbach G, Moreau C, Gandor F, Defebvre L, Devos D. Clinical syndromes: parkinsonian gait. Mov Disord. 2013;28:1552–9.
64. Backman L, Ginovart N, Dixon RA, Wahlin TB, Wahlin A, Halldin C, et al. Age-related cognitive deficits mediated by changes in the striatal dopamine system. Am J Psychiatry. 2000;157:635–7.
65. Brauer SG, Woollacott MH, Lamont R, Clewett S, O'Sullivan J, Silburn P, et al. Single and dual task gait training in people with Parkinson's disease: a protocol for a randomised controlled trial. BMC Neurol. 2011;11:90–4.
66. Baker K, Rochester L, Nieuwboer A. The immediate effect of attentional, auditory, and a combined cue strategy on gait during single and dual tasks in Parkinson's disease. Arch Phys Med Rehabil. 2007;88:1593–600.
67. Brown RG, Marsden CD. Dual task performance and processing resources in normal subjects and patients with Parkinson's disease. Brain. 1991;114:215–31.
68. Lohnes C, Earhart G. The impact of attentional, auditory, and combined cues on walking during single and cognitive dual tasks in Parkinson disease. Gait Posture. 2011;33:478–83.
69. Wild LB, Balardin JB, Lima DB, Rizzi L, Oliveira HB, Rieder CRM, et al. Characterization of cognitive and motor performance during dual-tasking in healthy older adults and patients with Parkinson's disease. J Neurol. 2013;20:580–9.
70. Foster ER, Hershey T. Everyday executive function is associated with activity participation in Parkinson disease without dementia. OTJR (Thorofare N J). 2011;31:16–22.
71. Mohlman J, Chazin D, Georgescu B. Feasibility and acceptance of a nonpharmacological cognitive remediation intervention for patients with Parkinson disease. J Geriatr Psychiatry Neurol. 2011;24:91–7.
72. Kelly VE, Eusterbrock AJ, Shumway-Cook A. The effects of instructions on dual-task walking and cognitive task performance in people with Parkinson's disease. Parkinsons Dis. 2012;2012:671261.
73. Montero-Odasso M, Verghese J, Beauchet O, Hausdorff JM. Gait and cognition: a complementary approach to understanding brain function and the risk of falling. JAGS. 2012;60:2127–36.
74. Stern Y. Cognitive reserve. Neuropsychologia. 2009;47:2015–28.
75. Jacobs JV, Dimitrova DM, Nutt JG, Horak FB. Can stooped posture explain multidirectional postural instability in patients with Parkinson's disease? Exp Brain Res. 2005;166:78–88.
76. Almeida QJ, Frank JS, Roy EA, Jenkins ME, Spaulding S, Patla AE, et al. An evaluation of sensorimotor integration during locomotion toward a target in Parkinson's disease. Neuroscience. 2005;134:283–93.
77. Jacobs JV, Horak FB. Abnormal proprioceptive-motor integration contributes to hypometric postural responses of subjects with Parkinson's disease. Neuroscience. 2006;141:999–1009.
78. Li F, Harmer P, Fitzgerald K, Eckstrom E, Stock R, Galver J, et al. Tai chi and postural stability in patients with Parkinson's disease. N Engl J Med. 2012;366:511–19.
79. Williams DR, Watt HC, Lees AJ. Predictors of falls and fractures in bradykinetic rigid syndromes: a retrospective study. J Neurol Neurosurg Psychiatry. 2006;77:468–73.
80. Morris ME, Menz HB, McGinley JL, Huxham FE, Murphy AT, Iansek R, et al. Falls and mobility in Parkinson's disease: protocol for a randomised controlled clinical trial. BMC Neurol. 2011;31:93–8.

81. Ebersbach G, Gunkel M. Posturography reflects clinical imbalance in Parkinson's disease. Mov Disord. 2011;26:241–6.
82. Ganesan M, Pal PK, Gupta A, Sathyaprabha TN. Dynamic posturography in evaluation of balance in patients of Parkinson's disease with normal pull test: concept of a diagonal pull test. Parkinsonism Relat Disord. 2010;16:595–9.
83. Ickenstein GW, Ambach H, Klöditz A, Koch H, Isenmann S, Reichmann H, et al. Static posturography in aging and Parkinson's disease. Front Aging Neurosci. 2012;6:20–8.
84. Valkovic P, Abrahámová D, Hlavacka F, Benetin J. Static posturography and infraclinical postural instability in early-stage Parkinson's disease. Mov Disord. 2009;24:1713–14.
85. Błaszczyk JW, Orawiec R. Assessment of postural control in patients with Parkinson's disease: sway ratio analysis. Hum Mov Sci. 2011;30:396–404.
86. Oude Nijhuis LB, Allum JH, Nanhoe-Mahabier W, Bloem BR. Influence of perturbation velocity on balance control in Parkinson's disease. PLoS One. 2014;9(1), e86650.
87. Chastan N, Debono B, Maltête D, Weber J. Discordance between measured postural instability and absence of clinical symptoms in Parkinson's disease patients in the early stages of the disease. Mov Disord. 2008;23:366–72.
88. Nardone A, Schieppati M. Balance in Parkinson's disease under static and dynamic conditions. Mov Disord. 2006;21:1515–20.
89. Barbosa A, Souza CO, Francato DV, Chen J, Chien HF, Barbosa ER, et al. Sensory-cognitive-motor interaction on postural balance in patients with Parkinson's disease. Arq Neuropsiquiatr. 2015;73:906–12.
90. Bloem BR, Marinus J, Almeida Q, Dibble L, Nieuwboer A, Post B, et al. Movement Disorders Society Rating Scales Committee. Measurement instruments to assess posture, gait, and balance in Parkinson's disease: critique and recommendations. Mov Disord. 2016. doi:10.1002/mds.26572.
91. Voos MC, Custódio EB, Malaquias Jr J. Relationship of executive function and educational status with functional balance in older adults. J Geriatr Phys Ther. 2011;34:11–8.
92. Souza Cde O, Voos MC, Francato DV, Chien HF, Barbosa ER. Influence of educational status on executive function and functional balance in individuals with Parkinson disease. Cogn Behav Neurol. 2013;26:6–13.
93. Dibble LE, Hale TF, Marcus RL, Droge J, Gerber JP, LaStayo PC. High-intensity resistance training amplifies muscle hypertrophy and functional gains in persons with Parkinson's disease. Mov Disord. 2006;21:1444–52.
94. Hirsch MA, Toole T, Maitland CG, Rider RA. The effects of balance training and high intensity resistance training on persons with idiopathic Parkinson's disease. Arch Phys Med Rehabil. 2003;84:1109–17.
95. Gracies JM. Neurorehabilitation in parkinsonian syndromes. Rev Neurol (Paris). 2010;166:196–212.
96. Morris ME. Movement disorders in people with Parkinson disease: a model for physical therapy. Phys Ther. 2000;80:578–97.
97. Al-Jarrah M, Jamous M, Al Zailaey K, Bweir SO. Endurance exercise training promotes angiogenesis in the brain of chronic/progressive mouse model of Parkinson's disease. NeuroRehabilitation. 2010;26:369–73.
98. Cadet P, Zhu W, Mantione K, Rymer M, Dardik I, Reisman S, et al. Cyclic exercise induces anti-inflammatory signal molecule increases in the plasma of Parkinson's patients. Int J Mol Med. 2003;12:485–92.
99. Wu SY, Wang TF, Yu L, Jen CJ, Chuang JI, Wu FS, et al. Running exercise protects the substantia nigra dopaminergic neurons against inflammation-induced degeneration via the activation of BDNF signaling pathway. Brain Behav Immun. 2011;25:135–46.
100. Lau YS, Patki G, Das-Panja K, Le WD, Ahmad SO. Neuroprotective effects and mechanisms of exercise in a chronic mouse model of Parkinson's disease with moderate neurodegeneration. Eur J Neurosci. 2011;33:1264–74.
101. Tajiri N, Yasuhara T, Shingo T, et al. Exercise exerts neuroprotective effects on Parkinson's disease model of rats. Brain Res. 2010;1310:200–7.

102. Cotman CW, Berchtold NC. Exercise: a behavioral intervention to enhance brain health and plasticity. Trends Neurosci. 2002;25:295–301.
103. Howells DW, Porritt MJ, Wong JY, Batchelor PE, Kalnins R, Hughes AJ, et al. Reduced BDNF mRNA expression in the Parkinson's disease substantia nigra. Exp Neurol. 2000;166:127–35.
104. Smith AD, Zigmond MJ. Can the brain be protected through exercise? Lessons from an animal model of parkinsonism. Exp Neurol. 2003;184:31–9.
105. Ahlskog JE. Does vigorous exercise have a neuroprotective effect in Parkinson disease? Neurology. 2011;77:288–94.
106. Petzinger GM, Fisher BE, McEwen S, Beeler JA, Walsh JP, Jakowec MW. Exercise-enhanced neuroplasticity targeting motor and cognitive circuitry in Parkinson's disease. Lancet Neurol. 2013;12:716–26.
107. Shu HF, Yang T, Yu SX, Huang HD, Jiang LL, Gu JW, et al. Aerobic exercise for Parkinson's disease: a systematic review and meta-analysis of randomized controlled trials. PLoS One. 2014;9, e100503.
108. Brienesse LA, Emerson MN. Effects of resistance training for people with Parkinson's disease: a systematic review. J Am Med Dir Assoc. 2013;14:236–41.
109. Reynolds GO, Otto MW, Ellis TD, Cronin-Golomb A. The therapeutic potential of exercise to improve mood, cognition, and sleep in Parkinson's disease. Mov Disord. 2016;31:23–38.
110. Frazzitta G, Balbi P, Maestri R, Bertotti G, Boveri N, Pezzoli G. The beneficial role of intensive exercise on Parkinson disease progression. Am J Phys Med Rehabil. 2013;92:523–32.
111. Earhart GM. Dance as therapy for individuals with Parkinson disease. Eur J Phys Rehabil Med. 2009;45:231–8.
112. Blandy LM, Beevers WA, Fitzmaurice K, Morris ME. Therapeutic argentine tango dancing for people with mild Parkinson's disease: a feasibility study. Front Neurol. 2015;6:122–7.
113. Duncan RP, Earhart GM. Are the effects of community-based dance on Parkinson disease severity, balance, and functional mobility reduced with time? A 2-year prospective pilot study. J Altern Complement Med. 2014;20:757–63.
114. Duncan RP, Earhart GM. Randomized controlled trial of community-based dancing to modify disease progression in Parkinson disease. Neurorehabil Neural Repair. 2012;26:132–43.
115. Tomlinson CL, Patel S, Meek C, Clarke CE, Stowe R, Shah L. Physiotherapy versus placebo or no intervention in Parkinson's disease. Cochrane Database Syst Rev. 2012;7, CD002817.
116. Bisson E, Contant B, Sveistrup H, Lajoie Y. Functional balance and dual-task reaction times in older adults are improved by virtual reality and biofeedback training. Cyberpsychol Behav. 2007;10:16–23.
117. Mirelman A, Maidan I, Deutsch JE. Virtual reality and motor imagery: promising tools for assessment and therapy in Parkinson's disease. Mov Disord. 2013;28:1597–608.
118. Mirelman A, Maidan I, Herman T, Deutsch JE, Giladi N, Hausdorff JM. Virtual reality for gait training: can it induce motor learning to enhance complex walking and reduce fall risk in patients with Parkinson's disease? J Gerontol A Biol Sci Med Sci. 2011;66:234–40.
119. Sewall GK, Jiang J, Ford CN. Clinical evaluation of Parkinson's-related dysphonia. Laryngoscope. 2006;116:1740–4.
120. Maillet A, Krainik A, Debu B, Tropres I, Lagrange C, Thobois S, et al. Levodopa effects on hand and speech movements in patients with Parkinson's disease: a fMRI study. PLoS One. 2012;7, e46541.
121. Mahler LA, Ramig LO, Fox C. Evidence-based treatment of voice and speech disorders in Parkinson disease. Curr Opin Otolaryngol Head Neck Surg. 2015;23:209–15.
122. Wight S, Miller N. Lee Silverman voice treatment for people with Parkinson's: audit of outcomes in a routine clinic. Int J Lang Commun Disord. 2015;50:2015–25.
123. Müller J, Wenning GK, Verny M, McKee A, Chaudhuri KR, Jellinger K, et al. Progression of dysarthria and dysphagia in postmortem-confirmed parkinsonian disorders. Arch Neurol. 2001;58:259–64.
124. Skodda S, Gronheit W, Mancinelli N, Schlegel U. Progression of voice and speech impairment in the course of Parkinson's disease: a longitudinal study. Parkinsons Dis. 2013;2013:389195.

125. Dias AE, Barbosa MT, Limongi JCP, Barbosa ER. Speech disorders did not correlate with age at onset of Parkinson's disease. Arq Neuro-Psiquiatr. 2016;74:117–21.
126. Atkinson-Clement C, Sadat J, Pinto S. Behavioral treatments for speech in Parkinson's disease: meta-analyses and review of the literature. Neurodegen Dis Manag. 2015;5:233–48.
127. Dias AE, Limongi JCP, Hsing WT, Barbosa ER. Digital inclusion for telerehabilitation speech in Parkinson's disease. J Parkinsons Dis. 2013;3:141.
128. Constantinescu G, Theodoros D, Russell T, Ward E, Wilson S, Wootton R. Treating disordered speech and voice in Parkinson's disease online: a randomized controlled non-inferiority trial. Int J Lang Commun Disord. 2011;46:1–16.
129. Molini-Avejonas DR, Rondon-Melo S, Amato CA, Samelli AG. A systematic review of the use of telehealth in speech language and hearing sciences. J Telemed Telecare. 2015;21:367–76.
130. Darling M, Huber JE. Changes to articulatory kinematics in response to loudness cues in individuals with Parkinson's disease. J Speech Lang Hear Res. 2011;54:1247–59.
131. Horstink M, Tolosa E, Bonuccelli U, Deuschl G, Friedman A, Kanovsky P, et al. Review of the therapeutic management of Parkinson's disease. Report of a joint task force of the European federation of neurological societies and the movement disorder society–European section. Part I: early (uncomplicated) Parkinson's disease. Eur J Neurol. 2006;13:1170–85.
132. Clarke C, Sullivan T, Mason A, Ford B, Nicholl D, Pamham J, et al. National Collaborating Centre for Chronic Conditions (Great Britain). Parkinson's disease: national clinical guideline for diagnosis and management in primary and secondary care. Royal College of Physicians, 2006.
133. Kalf H, de Swart B, Bonnier-Baars M, Kanters J, Hofman M, Kocken J, et al. Guidelines for speech-language therapy in Parkinson's disease—Concept translation parkinsonnet—NPF 2011;1–132.
134. Miller N. Speech, voice and language in Parkinson's disease: changes and interventions. Neurodegen Dis Manage. 2012;2:279–89.
135. Cleary RA, Poliakoff E, Galpin A, Dick JPR, Holler J. An investigation of co-speech gesture production during action description in Parkinson's disease. Parkinsonism Relat Disord. 2011;17:753–6.
136. Pell MD, Monetta L. How Parkinson's disease affects non-verbal communication and language processing. Lang Lingu Compass. 2008;2:739–59.
137. Rajaei A, Fereshteh A, Seyed AA, Ahmad C, Nilforoush MH, Taheri M, et al. The association between saliva control, silent saliva penetration, aspiration, and videofluoroscopic findings in Parkinson's disease patients. Adv Biomed Res. 2015;4:108.
138. Felix VN, Corrêa SMA, Soares RJ. A therapeutic maneuver for oropharyngeal dysphagia in patients with Parkinson disease. Clinics. 2008;63:661–6.
139. Suttrup I, Warnecke T. Dysphagia in Parkinson's disease. Dyphagia. 2016;31:24–32.
140. Warnecke T, Hamacher C, Oelenberg S, Dziewas R. Off and on-state assessment of swallowing function in Parkinson's disease. Parkinsonism Relat Disord. 2014;20:1033–4.
141. Paik NJ, Lorenzo CT. Dysphagia treatment & management: approach considerations. 2016. http://emedicine.medscape.com/article/2212409-treatment. Accessed 16 Apr 2016.
142. Troche MS, Brandimore AE, Foote KD, Okun MS. Swallowing and deep Brain stimulation in Parkinson's disease: a systematic review. Parkinsonism Relat Disord. 2013;19:783–8.
143. Michou E, Baijens L, Rofes L, Cartgena PS, Clavé P. Oropharyngeal swallowing in Parkinson's disease: revisited. Int J Speech Lang Pathol Audiol. 2013;1:76–88.
144. Crary MA. Treatment for adults. In: Crary MA, Groher ME, editors. Dysphagia: clinical management in adults and children. St. Louis: Elsevier/Mosby; 2009. p. 275–307.
145. Dand P, Sakel M. The management of drooling in motor neuron disease. Int J Palliat Nurs. 2010;16:560–4.
146. Srivanitchapoom P, Pandey S, Hallett M. Drooling in Parkinson's disease: a review. Parkinsonism Relat Disord. 2014;20:1109–18.
147. Sung HY, Kim JS, Lee KS, Kim YI, Song IU, Chung SW, et al. The prevalence and patterns of pharyngoesophageal dysmotility in patients with early stage Parkinson's disease. Mov Disord. 2010;25:2361–8.

148. Kalf JG, Munneke M, van den Engel-Hoek L, de Swart BJ, Borm GF, Bloem BR, Zwarts MJ. Pathophysiology of diurnal drooling in Parkinson's disease. Mov Disord. 2011;26:1670–6.
149. Sturkenboom IH, Graff MJ, Hendriks JC, Veenhuizen Y, Munneke M, Bloem BR, et al. Efficacy of occupational therapy for patients with Parkinson's disease: a randomised controlled trial. Lancet Neurol. 2014;13:557–66.
150. Monticone M, Ambrosini E, Laurini A, Rocca B, Foti C. In-patient multidisciplinary rehabilitation for Parkinson's disease: a randomized controlled trial. Mov Disord. 2015;30:1050–8.
151. Sturkenboom IH, Nijhuis-van der Sanden MW, Graff MJ. A process evaluation of a home-based occupational therapy intervention for Parkinson's patients and their caregivers performed alongside a randomized controlled trial. Clin Rehabil. 2015. doi:10.1177/0269215515622038.
152. Foster ER. Instrumental activities of daily living performance among people with Parkinson's disease without dementia. Am J Occup Ther. 2014;68:353–62.
153. Lidde J, Eagles R. Moderate evidence exists for occupational therapy-related interventions for people with Parkinson's disease in physical activity training, environmental cues and individualised programmes promoting personal control and quality of life. Aust Occup Ther J. 2014;61:287–8.
154. Sturkenboom IHWM, Thijssen MCE, Gons-van Elsacker JJ, Jansen IJH, Maasda A, Schulten M, et al. Guidelines for occupational therapy in Parkinson's disease rehabilitation. ParkinsonNet/NPF: Nijmegen/Miami; 2011.
155. Clarke CE, Patel S, Ives N, Rick CE, Dowling F, Woolley R, et al. Physiotherapy and occupational therapy vs no therapy in mild to moderate Parkinson disease: a randomized clinical trial. JAMA Neurol. 2016;73:291–9.
156. Foster ER, Bedekar M, Tickle-Degnen L. Systematic review of the effectiveness of occupational therapy-related interventions for people with Parkinson's disease. Am J Occup Ther. 2014;68:39–49.
157. Rao AK. Enabling functional independence in Parkinson's disease: update on occupational therapy intervention. Mov Disord. 2010;25(Suppl1):S146–51.
158. Murphy S, Tickle-Degnen L. The effectiveness of occupational therapy-related treatments for persons with Parkinson's disease: a meta-analytic review. Am J Occup Ther. 2001;55:385–92.
159. Ransmayr G. Physical, occupational, speech and swallowing therapies and physical exercise in Parkinson's disease. J Neural Transm (Vienna). 2011;118:773–81.
160. Dontje ML, de Greef MH, Speelman AD, van Nimwegen M, Krijnen WP, Stolk RP, et al. Quantifying daily physical activity and determinants in sedentary patients with Parkinson's disease. Parkinsonism Relat Disord. 2013;19:878–82.
161. Abbruzzese G, Marchese R, Avanzino L, Pelosin E. Rehabilitation for Parkinson's disease: current outlook and future challenges. Parkinsonism Relat Disord. 2016;22(Suppl1):S60–4.
162. Oguh O, Videnovic A. Inpatient management of Parkinson disease: current challenges and future directions. Neurohospitalist. 2012;2:28–35.
163. Proud EL, Miller KJ, Martin CL, Morris ME. Upper-limb assessment in people with Parkinson disease: is it a priority for therapists, and which assessment tools are used? Physiother Can. 2013;65:309–16.
164. Proud EL, Miller KJ, Bilney B, Balachandran S, McGinley JL, Morris ME. Evaluation of measures of upper limb functioning and disability in people with Parkinson disease: a systematic review. Arch Phys Med Rehabil. 2015;96:540–51.
165. Skinner JW, Lee HK, Roemmich RT, Amano S, Hass CJ. Execution of activities of daily living in persons with Parkinson disease. Med Sci Sports Exerc. 2015;47:1906–12.
166. Pitts DG, O'Brien SP. Splinting the hand to enhance motor control and brain plasticity. Top Stroke Rehabil. 2008;15:456–67.
167. Coelho M, Marti MJ, Tolosa E, Ferreira JJ, Valldeoriola F, Rosa M, et al. Late-stage Parkinson's disease: the Barcelona and Lisbon cohort. J Neurol. 2010;257:1524–32.
168. Aarsland D, Brønnick K, Fladby T. Mild cognitive impairment in Parkinson's disease. Curr Neurol Neurosci Rep. 2011;11:371–8.
169. Leung IH, Walton CC, Hallock H, Lewis SJ, Valenzuela M, Lampit A. Cognitive training in Parkinson disease: a systematic review and meta-analysis. Neurology. 2015;85:1843–51.

170. Ransmayr G. Cognitive impairment in Parkinson's disease. Psychiatr Danub. 2015; 27:458–61.
171. Nasreddine ZS, Phillips NA, Bédirian V, Charbonneau S, Whitehead V, Collin I, et al. The Montreal Cognitive Assessment, MoCA: a brief screening tool for mild cognitive impairment. J Am Geriatr Soc. 2005;53:695–9.
172. Chou KL, Amick MM, Brandt J, Camicioli R, Frei K, Gitelman D, et al. A recommended scale for cognitive screening in clinical trials of Parkinson's disease. Mov Disord. 2010;25:2501–7.
173. Folstein MF, Folstein SE, McHugh PR. Mini-mental state. A practical method for grading the cognitive state of patients for the clinician. J Psychiatry Res. 1975;12:189–98.
174. Lawton M, Kasten M, May MT, Mollenhauer B, Schaumburg M, Liepelt-Scarfone I, et al. Validation of conversion between mini-mental state examination and Montréal cognitive assessment. Mov Disord. 2016;31:593–6.
175. Domingos JM, Godinho C, Dean J, Coelho M, Pinto A, Bloem BR, et al. Cognitive impairment in fall-related studies in Parkinson's disease. J Parkinsons Dis. 2015;5:453–69.
176. Sturm W. Cognitive training in Parkinson disease: cognition-specific vs nonspecific computer training. Neurology. 2015;84:104.
177. Lawrence BJ, Gasson N, Kane R, Bucks RS, Loftus AM. Activities of daily living, depression, and quality of life in Parkinson's disease. PLoS One. 2014;15(9), e102294.
178. Choi Y, Park S, Cho KH, Chun SY, Park EC. A change in social activity affect cognitive function in middle-aged and older Koreans: analysis of a Korean longitudinal study on aging (2006–2012). Int J Geriatr Psychiatry. 2016;31(8):912–19. doi:10.1002/gps.4408.
179. Jansa J, Aragon A. Living with Parkinson's and the emerging role occupational therapy. Parkinsons Dis. 2015;2015:196303.
180. Law M, Baptiste S, Mc Coll M, Opzoomer A, Polatajko H, Pollock N. The Canadian occupational performance measure: an outcome measure for occupational therapy. Can J Occup Ther. 1990;57:82–7.
181. The Cure Parkinson's Trust. 2010. http://www.parkinsons.org.uk/content/parkinsons-self-assessment-tool. Accessed 3 Mar 2016.
182. Bhidayasiri R, Jitkritsadakul O, Boonrod N, Sringean J, Calne SM, Hattori N, et al. What is the evidence to support home environmental adaptation in Parkinson's disease? A call for multidisciplinary interventions. Parkinsonism Relat Disord. 2015;21:1127–32.
183. Demeulemeester F, De Letter M, Miatton M, Santens P. Quality of life in patients with PD and their caregiving spouses: a view from both sides. Clin Neurol Neurosurg. 2015;139:24–8.
184. Navarta-Sánchez MV, Senosiain García JM, Riverol M, Ursúa Sesma ME, Díaz de Cerio Ayesa S, Anaut Bravo S, et al. Factors influencing psychosocial adjustment and quality of life in Parkinson patients and informal caregivers. Qual Life Res. 2016;25(8):1959–68. doi:10.1007/s11136-015-1220-3.
185. Ricciardi L, Pomponi M, Demartini B, Ricciardi D, Morabito B, Bernabei R, et al. Emotional awareness, relationship quality, and satisfaction in patients with Parkinson's Disease and their spousal caregivers. J Nerv Ment Dis. 2015;203:646–9.
186. Yang WC, Wang HK, Wu RM, Lo CS, Lin KH. Home-based virtual reality balance training and conventional balance training in Parkinson's disease: a randomized controlled trial. J Formos Med Assoc. 2015. doi:10.1016/j.jfma.2015.07.012.
187. Cipresso P, Albani G, Serino S, Pedroli E, Pallavicini F, Mauro A, et al. Virtual multiple errands test (VMET): a virtual reality-based tool to detect early executive functions deficit in Parkinson's disease. Front Behav Neurosci. 2014;8:405.
188. Su KJ, Hwang WJ, Wu CY, Fang JJ, Leong IF, Ma HI. Increasing speed to improve arm movement and standing postural control in Parkinson's disease patients when catching virtual moving balls. Gait Posture. 2014;39:65–9.
189. Shine JM, Matar E, Ward PB, Frank MJ, Moustafa AA, Pearson M, et al. Freezing of gait in Parkinson's disease is associated with functional decoupling between the cognitive control network and the basal ganglia. Brain. 2013;136:3671–81.

190. Griffin H, Greenlaw R, Limousin P, Bhatia K, Quinn N, Jahanshahi M. The effect of real and virtual visual cues on walking in Parkinson's disease. J Neurol. 2011;258:991–1000.
191. Yen CY, Lin KH, Hu MH, Wu RM, Lu TW, Lin CH. Effects of virtual reality-augmented balance training on sensory organization and attentional demand for postural control in people with Parkinson disease: a randomized controlled trial. Phys Ther. 2011;91:862–74.
192. Albani G, Raspelli S, Carelli L, Morganti F, Weiss PL, Kizony R, et al. Executive functions in a virtual world: a study in Parkinson's disease. Stud Health Technol Inform. 2010;154:92–6.
193. Davidsdottir S, Wagenaar R, Young D, Cronin-Golomb A. Impact of optic flow perception and egocentric coordinates on veering in Parkinson's disease. Brain. 2008;131:2882–93.
194. Albani G, Pignatti R, Bertella L, Priano L, Semenza C, Molinari E, et al. Common daily activities in the virtual environment: a preliminary study in parkinsonian patients. Neurol Sci. 2002;23 Suppl 2:S49–50.

Atypical Parkinsonism

3

Orlando Graziani Povoas Barsottini,
Carolina de Oliveira Souza, Giovana Diaferia,
and Alberto J. Espay

Introduction

Approximately 15–25 % of patients initially diagnosed with Parkinson's disease (PD) may in fact have an alternative underlying pathological condition such as an atypical form of parkinsonism (ADP; previously referred to as "Parkinson-plus syndrome"). These patients may present with symptoms and signs uncommon for PD and their response to high doses of levodopa is poor [1, 2]. ATPs include progressive supranuclear palsy (PSP), multiple system atrophy (MSA), corticobasal degeneration (CBD), and dementia with Lewy bodies (DLB). Currently, this group also includes rare familial APDs associated with mutations in the microtubule-associated protein tau (*MAPT*) and progranulin (*PRGN*) genes, chromosome 9 open reading frame 72 (*C9ORF72*), chromatin modifying protein 2B (*CHMP2B*), and transactive DNA-binding protein (*TARDBP*) [3]. However, these rare forms of APD will not be dealt with in this chapter. Only the more common PSP, MSA, and CBD will be addressed here. Please note that, lacking reliable biomarkers, the definitive diagnosis of these disorders can only be made on pathological examination of the brain of affected patients [1, 2].

O.G.P. Barsottini, M.D., Ph.D. (✉)
Department of Neurology, Universidade Federal de São Paulo, São Paulo, Brazil
e-mail: orlandobarsottini@gmail.com

C. de Oliveira Souza, P.T., M.Sc.
Department of Neurology, Hospital das Clínicas da Faculdade de Medicina da Universidade de São Paulo, São Paulo, Brazil
e-mail: souzaco@usp.br

G. Diaferia, S.L.P., M.Sc.
Department of Neurology, Universidade Federal de São Paulo, São Paulo, Brazil
e-mail: gidiaferia@hotmail.com

A.J. Espay, M.D., M.Sc.
Department of Neurology, University of Cincinnati, Cincinnati, OH 45267, USA
e-mail: aespay@gmail.com

© Springer International Publishing Switzerland 2017
H.F. Chien, O.G.P. Barsottini (eds.), *Movement Disorders Rehabilitation*,
DOI 10.1007/978-3-319-46062-8_3

Multiple System Atrophy

Multiple system atrophy is a sporadic neurodegenerative disease characterized by the association of parkinsonism, cerebellar, pyramidal, and autonomic symptoms [2]. The estimated annual prevalence of MSA is 0.6 per 100,000 people per year, reaching 3 per 100,000 in people aged over 50 years [4, 5]. The mean survival rate is around 6–7 years. Nearly 20 years after the introduction of the term MSA, abundant glial cytoplasmic inclusions containing alpha-synuclein have been described as disease markers. Because of similar protein aggregation in PD and DLB, MSA is classified within the group of neurological disorders termed "synucleinopathies" [6]. The diagnostic criteria for MSA were first formulated in 1999 and a specific evaluation scale was developed in 2004 (the Unified Multiple System Atrophy Rating Scale [UMSARS]) [7]. *SNCA* gene encodes for alpha-synuclein protein and *SNCA* variants may be risk factors for developing MSA [8]. Recently, heterozygous variants of the coenzyme Q2 4-hydroxybenzoate polyprenyltransferase (*COQ2*) gene were identified as being a cause of familial MSA in Japan [9].

Multiple system atrophy with predominantly parkinsonian features (previous nomenclature, *striatonigral degeneration*) is referred to as MSA-P, and with predominantly cerebellar symptoms (*olivopontocerebellar atrophy*) as MSA-C [1, 2]. There is a predominance of autonomic symptoms (previous eponym, *Shy-Drager syndrome*) in most cases early on or with disease progression. Patients may initially respond to levodopa, but similar to other forms of APD, the response generally disappears with disease progression. Dysautonomia is mainly characterized by erectile dysfunction in men, urinary incontinence or retention in women, postural hypotension, constipation, and excessive sweating [1, 2, 6]. Rapid eye movement (REM) sleep behavior disorder is very common in MSA and may predate its onset as it does in PD. Dysarthria and, to a lesser extent, dysphagia, typically appear within the first year of the disease, and, in the presence of "cold blue hands" and anterocollis, they make the diagnosis more likely. Early overt cognitive dysfunction similar to that seen in other forms of APD is unusual, but neuropsychological assessments may reveal subclinical deficits in executive functions [1, 2, 6].

Patients with MSA may develop levodopa-induced dyskinesia soon after initiation of treatment. It is interesting to note that these dyskinesias typically involve the face and neck, but are rarely widespread [6].

Multiple system atrophy is pathologically characterized by neuronal loss and gliosis in the putamen, caudate nucleus, globus pallidus, substantia nigra, inferior olives, pontine nuclei, Purkinje cells, autonomic brainstem nuclei, intermediolateral cell columns of the spinal cord, and Onuf's nucleus. Although cytoplasmic inclusions may aggregate within neurons, they are characteristic in oligodendrocytes, leading to the suggestion that MSA might be considered a primary oligodendrogliopathy from a pathological standpoint [2, 8].

Brain MRI studies of patients with MSA-P reveal marked putaminal atrophy whereas patients with MSA-C show cerebellar, superior cerebellar peduncle, and pontine atropy, with a "hot cross bun" sign and increased signal abnormalities in the middle cerebellar penduncles (Fig. 3.1) [10]. Abnormal anal and urethral

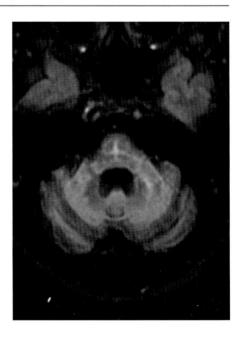

Fig. 3.1 Brain MRI with the "hot cross bun" sign in a patient with multiple system atrophy (cerebellar type)

sphincter electromyography may be due to degenerative changes in Onuf's nucleus of the spinal cord [6]. Cardiac scintigraphy with metaiodobenzylguanidine (MIBG) can be a useful cardiac autonomic marker for differentiating MSA from PD because it is abnormal in patients with PD. Studies of sleep disorders such as polysomnography can reveal REM behavior disorder, laryngeal stridor, sleep apnea, and excessive snoring, some of which may precede the onset of the motor features by several years. Other autonomic function studies such as the tilt table test may detect postural hypotension even in asymptomatic patients and should be obtained to fully document the extent of autonomic dysfunction when a diagnosis of MSA is suspected [1, 2, 6, 7].

Levodopa may have benefits in the early stage of the disease; however, its effectiveness wanes as the disease progresses [2]. Minocycline, a tetracycline with potential neuroprotective effect, did not change the disease course after 24 and 48 weeks of treatment in a randomized double-blind study (Minocycline European MSA Trial) [11]. Recent clinical trials (2013–2015) showed no benefits of treatment with lithium, rifampicin, riluzole, and rasagiline in patients with MSA [12].

Postural hypotension can be addressed with simple practical measures including a high-salt diet, increased fluid intake, use of thigh-high compression stockings and head-of-bed elevation during sleep. If these measures are not sufficiently effective, pharmacological measures include fludrocortisone (0.1–0.3 mg daily), midodrine (2.5–10 mg 3 times daily), and droxidopa (100–600 mg 3 times daily). Urinary incontinence is usually treated with oxybutynin (5–10 mg at bedtime), although its use may be associated with the magnification of any cognitive dysfunction. Constipation may be alleviated using laxatives and high-fiber foods. There are positive reports on the use of sildenafil for erectile dysfunction in patients with MSA [2, 6].

Progressive Supranuclear Palsy

Progressive supranuclear palsy, also called Steele–Richardson–Olszewski syndrome in honor of the three pioneers who identified this nosological entity, is a distinctive and probably underdiagnosed neurodegenerative syndrome. It is the second most common cause of degenerative parkinsonism after PD in most series [13, 14]. The "classic" PSP syndrome, also referred to as Richardson syndrome, is characterized by a higher level (frontal) gait impairment, ophthalmoparesis (predominantly downward gaze palsy without correction with oculocephalic maneuvers [supranuclear vertical gaze palsy]), frontal cognitive dysfunction, and (often tremorless) symmetrical, axial-predominant, posturally impaired parkinsonism with falls occurring within a year of symptom onset [2]. Retrocollis and apraxia of eyelid opening are focal/segmental dystonic manifestations that may be documented in PSP. A subset of patients develops bulbar as well as pseudobulbar manifestations, particularly pseudobulbar affect (emotional incontinence). The prevalence of PSP is age-dependent and estimated to be 6–10 % of the incidence of PD, or 6–7 cases per 100,000 people [15, 16]. PSP has a peak onset at the age of 63 years with no cases reported under the age of 40. The clinically probable diagnosis, which is the highest antemortem category of diagnostic certainty (definitive diagnosis can only be made at autopsy), is usually made 3.6–4.9 years after the onset of clinical signs [15].

There have been increasing clinical, neuroimaging, molecular pathology, and genetic insights into PSP in recent years. It is a tauopathy characterized by deposits of neurofibrillary tangles in the brain that are made of hyperphosphorylated microtubule-associated protein tau. The abnormal tau protein and neuropil threads accumulate in the subthalamic nucleus, globus pallidum, red nucleus, substantia nigra, striatum, pontine tegmentum, oculomotor nucleus, medulla, and dentate nucleus. Although a few familial cases with *MAPT* gene mutations have been reported, this disorder remains largely sporadic. A genome-wide association study has confirmed that the most common risk allele for PSP is the H1 haplotype of the *MAPT* gene [15–17].

In the adult human brain, tau protein has six isoforms formed by alternative splicing that are derived from a single gene. Disordered regulation of exon 10 splicing may therefore explain tau aggregation into neurofibrillary tangles in PSP and other tauopathies. The microtubule-binding domain contains either three 31 amino acid repeats (3R) or four 31 amino acid repeats (4R). In the normal adult brain, the ratio of 3R and 4R tau isoforms is similar. In PSP, it is at least 3:1 in favor of 4R tau [2, 15–17].

Similar histopathological findings can be seen in other forms of tauopathies (e.g., Guadeloupian parkinsonism), which complicates the pathological diagnosis of PSP. The most specific features are star-shaped astrocytic tufts and neurofibrillary tangles that are seen under light microscopy and strongly immunostain with tau antibodies [16, 17].

Progressive supranuclear palsy is frequently misdiagnosed as PD, and less than half of patients with pathologically proven PSP are diagnosed correctly as having PSP at presentation. The National Institute of Neurological Disorders and Stroke/Society for PSP (NINDS/SPSP) criteria detect disease in only 50–70 % of patients in the first 3 years after disease onset [18]. These diagnostic shortcomings may at least in part be due to the phenotypic diversity, grouped into six well-documented clinical PSP phenotypes, recognized through neuropathological studies [15, 16]

1. **Richardson's syndrome (RS)**: As described above, this is the "classic" clinical presentation of PSP.
2. **PSP parkinsonism (PSP-P)**: The PSP-P phenotype occurs in about one-third of cases and is a more indolent form with a PD-like levodopa-responsive presentation. This is the type most likely to be diagnosed as PD for the first 5 years, as falls and oculomotor abnormalities do not occur until at least that many years have passed.
3. **PSP pure akinesia with gait freezing (PSP-PAGF)**: This PSP phenotype is highly predictive of PSP-tau pathology. It occurs as a syndrome that includes progressive gait disturbance with start hesitation and subsequent freezing of gait, speech or writing in the absence of tremor, rigidity, dementia or eye movement abnormalities during the first 5 years of the disease.
4. **PSP progressive non-fluent aphasia (PSP-PNFA)**: It is characterized by non-fluent spontaneous speech with hesitancy, phonemic errors, and agrammatism. This language-based PSP presentation also includes the more recently identified syndrome "progressive apraxia of speech."
5. **PSP cerebellar**: Kanazawa et al. [19] described cerebellar involvement in PSP. They studied 22 consecutive Japanese patients with pathologically proven PSP and 3 patients developed cerebellar ataxia as the first major symptom.
6. **PSP corticobasal syndrome (PSP-CBS)**: It is characterized by progressive, asymmetrical, levodopa-unresponsive parkinsonism with ideomotor apraxia, cortical sensory loss, alien limb phenomenology, dystonia, and myoclonus of the most severely affected limb.

The most important MRI abnormalities in PSP patients are midbrain atrophy and superior peduncle atrophy (Fig. 3.2) [20]. The "humming bird" and "morning glory" signs have high specificity but rather low sensitivity [16, 17]. [^{18}F]-fluorodeoxyglucose (FDG) positron emission tomography (PET) studies in PSP patients show characteristic brain glucose hypometabolism in the mesial frontal and insular regions and in the midbrain [2].

There are no effective symptomatic or curative treatments for PSP. Poor or absent response to levodopa is one of the diagnostic criteria for PSP with marked or prolonged levodopa benefit being an exclusion criterion [2, 15, 16]. Serotoninergic drugs such as selective serotonin reuptake inhibitors, 5-hydroxytryptophan, and methysergide have no confirmed benefit in PSP, in addition to cholinergic drugs, such as acetylcholinesterase (AChE) inhibitors, and muscarinic agonists. Botulinum toxin may be helpful in PSP for treating dystonia such as retrocollis and apraxia of eyelid opening, reducing disability provoked by these symptoms [15]. A dextromethorphan/quinidine combination may be helpful among those who develop troublesome pseudobulbar affect. Recent clinical trials with tideglusib (an inhibitor of glycogen

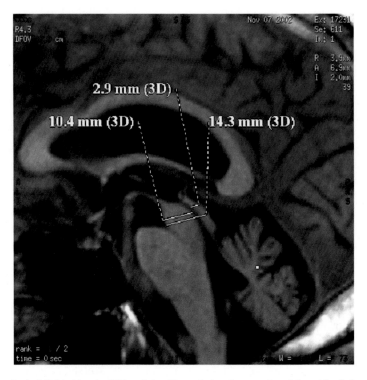

Fig. 3.2 Brain MRI (midsagittal T1-weighted image) showing atrophy of the midbrain in a patient with progressive supranuclear palsy

synthase kinase-3), davunetide intranasal spray (shown to promote microtubule stability and reduce tau phosphorylation), and high-dose coenzyme Q10 and rasagiline (1 mg/day) have failed to support clinical benefits [12].

Corticobasal Degeneration

Corticobasal degeneration (CBD) was first described in 1968 as a "corticodentatonigral degeneration with neuronal achromasia" [21] and is the leading cause of the so-called corticobasal syndrome (CBS). Given the heterogeneity of the clinical syndrome (CBS can be due to many etiologies, including CBD, but also Alzheimer's disease, frontotemporal lobar degeneration, and PSP) and the pathological syndrome (CBD can be associated with CBS, PSP syndrome, PNFA, and posterior cortical atrophy syndrome), the diagnosis of CBD/CBS may remain elusive during life [2]. Only 25–56 % of suspected CBS cases have been given pathological confirmation of CBD [22]. CBS typically presents in the sixth decade of life with markedly asymmetrical symptoms in the upper limbs, less commonly in the lower limbs. It is evenly distributed between the sexes and, owing to its rare occurrence, the exact prevalence of this syndrome is not known but is believed to be around 2 in 1,000,000 people [2, 23, 24]. It is a progressive disease with a survival span of about 7 years. The most common clinical signs and symptoms are asymmetrical levodopa-resistant parkinsonism with dystonia, myoclonus, and cortical signs, including cortical sensory loss, apraxia, and alien limb phenomenon in the most severely affected limb. Cognitive impairment tends to be less overt than in PSP but greater than in MSA. Other less common symptoms are abnormal eye movements (increased latency of saccades), postural instability, falls, abnormal gait, axial rigidity, and a high-amplitude tremor that is greater posturally when resting [2, 22, 23].

Corticobasal degeneration is characterized by the widespread deposition of hyperphosphorylated 4-repeat tau in neurons and glia, and neuronal degeneration in the frontotemporal cortex and substantia nigra. The hallmark feature is the astrocytic plaques that differentiate CBD from other 4R tauopathies, particularly PSP. Similar to PSP, CBD is associated with the H1 haplotype of the *MAPT* gene [24].

Neuropathological studies have shown that CBS may be due to Alzheimer's disease, PSP, and forms of frontotemporal dementia. Conversely, pathologically confirmed CBD cases may exhibit a range of phenotypes including CBS but also frontotemporal dementia, primary progressive aphasia (PNFA, in particular), and posterior cortical atrophy [2, 25].

Neuroimaging studies of CBS patients, including brain MRI and FDG-PET or SPECT, show asymmetrical frontoparietal atrophy and hypometabolism respectively [26]. Cerebrospinal fluid biomarkers have not yet been adequately studied in patients with CBS/CBD [22–24].

As with other forms of APD, there is a low yield in the symptomatic treatment available for CBS. There is generally no response to dopaminergic drugs, including levodopa at doses as high as 2 g/day. Myoclonus can be alleviated with clonazepam and/or valproate or levetiracetam. Focal arm dystonia may be alleviated with anticholinergic drugs or botulinum toxin [2]. Dementia can be treated with cholinesterase inhibitors, but the effectiveness of this approach remains unproven.

Physical Therapy in Parkinsonian Syndromes

There is scarce evidence on specific physical therapies in parkinsonian syndromes, such as PSP, MSA, and CBD. In most cases, long-term efficacy has not been reported. Patients with APD reviewed above can exhibit faster progression, less or no response to antiparkinsonian medications, and shorter survival compared with PD, all of which limit response to physiotherapy. Further controlled studies to provide guidance to physical therapists in the management of these diseases are lacking.

Below is a summary of the (largely anecdotal [case reports or case series]) studies investigating the effect of physical therapy to improve motor control in patients with PSP, MSA and CBD.

Physical Therapy in Progressive Supranuclear Palsy

Patients with PSP are usually referred for physical therapy (PT) to treat balance and gait problems with frequent falls. Gait training and movement strategies that are useful in PD may also be applicable in PSP and other APDs. Behaviorally, balance impairment in the mediolateral plane (i.e., sideways) is often seen in patients with

APDs, but not in patients with PD [27]. This is reflected by the distance between the feet during gait, which is typically normal (or even narrow) in PD, but widened in PSP and MSA. Estimating this stance width is difficult in clinical practice, without objective measures. Nevertheless, this mediolateral balance impairment can be revealed using two simple tests: (1) inability to perform tandem gait (one or more side steps being abnormal) [28]; and (2) self-report by patients who have lost the ability to ride a bicycle [29]. Both tests are useful for distinguishing PD from atypical parkinsonism, even in the early course of the disease [27].

Suteerawattananon et al. [30] described the rehabilitation of one patient (a 62-year-old man) diagnosed with PSP. His major problems were impaired balance and frequent, abrupt falls. His PT program included walking training, balance perturbation, and step training using body weight support with a treadmill. Training sessions lasted 1.5 h and took place 3 days a week for 8 weeks. Fall incidence, balance, and gait were assessed before, during, and after the program. The patient reported fewer falls during and after training. Balance and gait improved after training [30].

Steffen et al. [31] evaluated a 72-year-old man diagnosed with mixed PSP and CBS features after 6 years of disease. He had asymmetric limb apraxia, markedly impaired balance, and frequent falls during transitional movements. PT intervention included routine participation in a PD group exercise program (mat exercises and treadmill training) and intermittent participation in individual locomotor training on a treadmill. The exercise group met for 1 h, twice weekly. The individual treadmill sessions lasted 1 h, once weekly, for two 14-week periods during the follow-up period. Over a 2.5-year follow-up period, fall frequency decreased, and tests of functional balance showed improved stability (functional reach tests) and maintained balance function (Berg Balance Scale). Tests of walking performance showed only a slight decline. A four-wheeled walker was introduced and accepted by the patient early in the intervention period. With supervision, he remained ambulatory in the community with this wheeled walker. The authors concluded that PT, relying on locomotor training using a treadmill and a long-term exercise program of stretching and strengthening, may improve some dimensions of balance, slow the rate of gait decline, prevent progression to wheelchair dependence, and decrease the number of falls. Contrary to the expected decline in function, this patient maintained independent mobility beyond 2 years [31].

Steffen et al. [32] subsequently published a longer-term (10 years) follow-up in the same PSP/CBS patient. The falls (reported weekly over the study period by the patient and his wife) decreased from 1.9 falls per month in year 1 to 0.3 falls per month in year 10. Taken together, the functional data described in these reports with regard to mobility, balance, walking speed, falls, and endurance strongly suggest the importance of a regular and aggressive exercise program to prolong longevity, decrease the number of falls, and promote stability of function (including balance and ambulation) for a patient with suspected CBS/PSP syndrome [32].

It is known that people with PSP have difficulty suppressing the vestibulo-ocular reflex (VOR) [18]. The inability to generate saccades can compromise safe ambulation.

Anticipatory saccades normally occur in situations that involve changing the direction of walking [33] or before obstacle avoidance [34]. When saccades are not generated quickly, there is an increased risk for falling [35].

Rehabilitation strategies for PSP are likely to differ from those for PD because vertical gaze palsy is unique to PSP and has the potential to create additional balance and mobility problems. Therefore, the rehabilitation for PSP should involve "eye-movement training" in addition to balance and gait training.

Lindemann et al. [36], using dual-tasking paradigms to assess differences between patients with PSP who fell frequently and those who fell less often, found more ocular movement difficulties, decreased postural stability, and decreased cognition in the former than in the latter group. The frequent fallers demonstrated a significant increase in cadence and a decrease in step length compared with the infrequent fallers, but the groups did not differ significantly under dual tasking for maximal gait speed. These findings may reflect a first adaptation with dual tasking to produce safer walking by decreasing step length. A decrease in cadence was found to be the next adaptation, when needed. These findings also suggest that falls might result from cognitive and ocular dysfunction in addition to the parkinsonian features [36].

Zampieri et al. [37] investigated 19 adults with possible or probable PSP and postural instability. Balance training accompanied by eye movement and visual awareness exercises was compared with balance training alone. The gaze control was assessed using a vertical gaze fixation score and a gaze error index. Gaze control after the balance plus eye exercise significantly improved, whereas no significant improvement was observed for the group that received balance training alone [37].

Recently, Seamon et al. [38] described an intervention using a virtual gaming system to improve gait, postural control, and cognitive awareness to reduce falls and improve the quality of life for a patient with PSP. A 65-year-old woman with a 5-year disease duration and frequent falls, poor ability to visually track objects, axial rigidity, retropulsion, poor postural control, with reaching and cognitive decline was assessed. She was provided with the Xbox Kinect for 12 one-hour sessions over 6 weeks in an outpatient setting. The games were selected to challenge functional motor and cognitive tasks based on patient enjoyment. After the intervention with virtual reality the patient showed decreased falls and maintenance of scores on the Berg Balance Scale, Timed Up and Go (TUG), and 10-Meter Walk Tests above fall risk values. A decline in quality of life measures, PDQ-39 and Fear of Falling Avoidance Behavior Questionnaire, may be attributed to an increase in cognitive awareness of deficits promoted by the intervention structure. According to the authors, the implementation of a gaming intervention using a virtual gaming system is feasible for reducing fall risk and maintaining function and mobility when used in an outpatient setting [38].

In conclusion, these studies have suggested that a combination of balance/walk interventions [30–32, 37, 38] and eye movement training [37] may improve the functional performance of patients with PSP.

Physical Therapy in Multiple System Atrophy

Patients with MSA present not only a functional incapacity, but also a greater severity of motor symptoms compared with patients with PD [39]. They also exhibit muscle weakness [40] with subsequent impaired muscle performance [41] and loss of balance [39]. These factors contribute to an increased risk for falls. Clinical practice suggests that most patients might be poorly responsive to antiparkinsonian drugs. In this context, rehabilitation strategies may be helpful.

The beneficial effects of Tai Chi in the improvement of gait and posture in PD patients are well established in the literature [42–44]. Venglar [45] described the effects of an 8-week Tai Chi class on two patients: one with PD, the other MSA. Both patients demonstrated improved scores on the Activities-specific Balance Confidence Scale and the Functional Reach Test. One subject also demonstrated improved scores for the Timed Up and Go test. Both subjects reported subjective improvements in balance and balance awareness. This study indicated that Tai Chi might be a viable option for improving balance in patients with MSA [45].

Wedge [41] showed that a low to moderate intensity conventional resistance training program was able to improve the functional ability, balance, and muscle performance in a 68-year-old woman with a 2-year history of MSA. Examination included range of motion, muscle strength, motor control ambulation with and without assistive device, and determination of orthostatic hypotension. Functional Reach, TUG, timed single limb stance, and the Performance Oriented Mobility Assessment tests were used to assess safety, balance, and fall risk. Hypokinesia and festinating gait were observed during ambulation. Transfers from sitting to standing were functional, but compromised safety. Impairments of muscle performance were found at the ankle, knee, and hip. Low to moderate intensity, lower extremity resistance training was added (twice weekly) to an existing program of balance and flexibility exercises. Clinically meaningful gains were achieved in all functional measures, and the patient performed SLS for 10 s when previously unable. More importantly, she achieved her goal of remaining at home. The addition of resistance training to an existing program of balance and flexibility exercises did not cause any adverse effects and appears to have led to improvements in balance and functional ability [41].

Batista et al. [46] assessed quality of life, activities of daily living, motor symptoms, functional ability, and neuromuscular parameters in a patient with MSA. The program of resistance training with instability was performed twice a week during 24 weeks for a total of 48 sessions performed. The patient was tested and trained in the clinically "on" state (fully medicated) during the morning time within 1.5 h of taking his last dose of the dopaminergic drug. Each training session lasted between 40 and 50 min, and started with a 10-min warm-up on a bicycle ergometer (20–40 rpm). The resistance training with instability devices consisted of conventional external load lower-limb resistance training machines (i.e., leg press and plantar flexion) and free exercise (i.e., half-squat) with unstable devices (i.e., balance pad, dyna discs, balance discs, BOSU ball, and Swiss ball). The unstable devices were placed between the patient's base of support (i.e., the body area responsible for sustaining most of his body weight and/or on the point of force application) and the resistance training machines for each individual exercise. Progression with the unstable device was included in the training program from less unstable to more unstable. After the 6-month training, the patient's left and right quadriceps muscle cross-sectional areas and leg press one-repetition maximum increased by 6.4%, 6.8%, and 40% respectively; the TUG, sitting to standing transfer, dynamic balance, and activities of daily living improved by 33.3%, 28.6%, 42.3%, and 40.1% respectively; and the severity of motor symptoms and risk of falls decreased by 32% and 128.1% respectively. Most of the subscales of quality of life demonstrated improvements as well, varying from 13.0 to 100.0%. This study showed that resistance training may decrease the severity of motor symptoms and risk of falls, and improve functional ability, neuromuscular parameters, and quality of the life in patients with MSA [46].

Current treatment strategies for MSA focus on the control of neurogenic orthostatic hypotension (nOH) [47]. Patients with severe nOH suffer from debilitating symptoms that substantially impair their ability to complete activities of daily living and reduce their quality of life. A high incidence of fall-related fractures and trauma occurs in patients with severe nOH [48]. Classic nOH symptoms, such as orthostatic dizziness and syncope, and less appreciated symptoms, such as coat-hanger pain and cognitive impairment, can force patients to curtail activities that involve standing or walking [49]. In addition to pharmacological strategies (see above) [50] patients may be treated with physiotherapy[51]. Exercises, especially activities that are performed recumbent or in water, are encouraged to prevent deconditioning, which can exacerbate nOH [52]. However, patients should avoid exercising in the morning, when orthostatic symptoms are typically worse. Is also recommended that when changing position they should do so slowly to allow time for autonomic adaption. For instance, when going from a supine position to walking, patients should sit before standing and stand for several minutes before walking [53].

Physical Therapy in Corticobasal Syndrome
Early in the disease course, PT may help to improve or maintain mobility and help with assessing the need for assistive devices (e.g., walkers) to improve gait and decrease the risk for falls. Later in the disease course, involvement of physiotherapists is critical for home safety assessments and appropriate wheelchair provision (e.g., to prevent pressure ulcers) and to instruct caregivers on range of motion exercises.

To our knowledge, there are only two studies describing the effects of PT [54] and PT plus repetitive transcranial magnetic stimulation (rTMS) [55] in patients with CBS.

Kawahira et al. [54] studied the effect of repetitive facilitation exercise in a patient with CBS. This exercise included movements of each isolated finger using the stretch reflex and skin–muscle reflex and repetitive movements demanded in activities of daily living and manipulation of objects. To evaluate improvements in hand functions by repetitive facilitation exercise, 1-week repetitive facilitation exercise sessions for the hand were administered alternatively to the left or right hand. The number of finger taps by the hand increased during each 1-week repetitive facilitation exercise session for the hand, but did not increase during 1-week sessions without repetitive facilitation exercise. After 1 month of treatment, there was an improvement in activities of daily living, including wearing clothes, manipulating objects, and cooking. These results suggest that facilitation exercises and repetition movements in activities of daily living might aid recovery in patients with CBS [54].

Shehata et al. [55] investigated low-frequency repetitive transcranial magnetic stimulation (rTMS) as a therapeutic tool in CBS. Twenty-six patients with clinically probable CBS were followed for 12–18 months while receiving low-frequency rTMS combined with rehabilitation treatment and botulinum toxin injection in the affected dystonic limb. There was improvement in the UPDRS (measure of motor severity) and quality of life after 3 months of therapeutic interventions ($P<0.001$ and <0.05 respectively). No significant deterioration in cognitive function was detected over the study period. There was a reduction in the caregiver burden after 3 months of interventions ($P<0.01$); this improvement was maintained for up to 18 months. The authors concluded that the combined treatment approach was effective in improving quality of life and reducing the caregiver burden [55].

Demand for rehabilitation in this and other parkinsonian populations will increase, but more research is necessary to answer basic questions regarding the type and dosage of the above rehabilitation strategies.

Speech Therapy in APD

Multiple System Atrophy

Dysarthria and dysphagia are known to occur in MSA, PSP, and CBD [56]. Some studies report that the appearance of dysarthria during the first year of disease in patients with degenerative parkinsonism strongly suggests one of these disorders, most commonly MSA or PSP [57].

The response to levodopa is negligible. As a result, the multidisciplinary patient support through speech therapists, physiotherapists, occupational therapists, and nurses plays an important role in the treatment [58]. Speech and voice alterations are due to impairments in muscle control caused by central and, to a lesser extent, peripheral nervous system involvement [59]. The speech abnormalities of these disorders can be classified as hypokinetic, ataxic, hyperkinetic, spastic, and mixed [60]. To develop effective methods of speech therapy to improve the communication of patients, it is necessary, first, to classify the speech–language disorders into these *dysarthrophonia* categories.

A study conducted by Knopp et al. [61] characterized the disorders of speech and voice of five patients with MSA, with a mean age of 51.2 years. The symptoms of speech and voice appeared 1.1 years after the onset of motor symptoms. In all patients, dysarthrophonia was the mixed type, combining the hypokinetic components, ataxic and spastic, the former being predominant.

In the 1990s, Countryman et al. [62] examined the Lee Silverman Voice Treatment (LSVT), originally designed for PD patients, in two patients with MSA, with different outcomes for each, according to the predominance of parkinsonian or autonomic features. Thus, not only the classification of the type of dysarthrophonia is important, but also distinguishing the predominant symptoms.

In a classical description of 100 cases Wenning et al. [63] reported that dysarthria occurs in almost all patients with MSA confirmed post-mortem. Typically, voice and speech alterations that accompany APDs are different from those observed in PD, especially with regard to two specific points: gravity in relation to the duration of the disease and the type of dysarthrophonia. Quinn [64] suggests that a diagnostic indicator of MSA is the occurrence of more severe symptoms and faster speech deterioration than in PD. In PD, the average interval between the onset of motor symptoms and speech symptoms is 6.3 years [65]. The dysarthrophonia accompanying PD is classified as hypokinetic and the perceptual features are: monotone, articulatory imprecision, inadequate breaks, speech jets, hoarse and breathy voice, and speech rate alteration [66]. However, the description of dysarthrophonia of MSA has been different from that of PD: these patients have excess hoarseness, intermittent baseline emission (lowest frequency of the vocal range) and decreased speech rate [67]. In a study of 46 MSA patients, Kluin et al. [68] concluded that the type of dysarthrophonia that characterizes this population is the mixed type, with the combination of hypokinetic and ataxic–spastic components: hypokinetic in 48 %, ataxic in 35 %, and spastic in 11 %. Rehman [69] also reported mixed dysarthrophonia with hypokinetic and ataxic–spastic components.

Higo et al. [70] investigated the swallowing function of 21 patients with MSA-C using videofluoroscopy (VF). Swallowing function in the oral phase became gradually disturbed during the progression of MSA. Delayed bolus transport from the oral cavity to the pharynx had already been seen in 50 % of the patients within 1–3 years following disease onset (the early stage of the disease), and it was seen in more than 85 % of the patients within more than 7 years following disease onset (the late stage of the disease). Bolus holding in the oral cavity was slightly disturbed in the early stage of the disease, but it was seen in 57 % of the patients in the late stage of the disease. This study showed that parkinsonism is related to swallowing dysfunction in MSA, but cerebellar dysfunction also affects coordination of the tongue; bolus transport in the oral cavity was disturbed in the early stage of disease. Progression of cerebellar dysfunction and overlapped parkinsonism worsened tongue movements, and in the late stage of the disease, swallowing function of the oral phase (bolus transport and bolus holding) was remarkably disturbed. Swallowing function in the pharyngeal phase did not significantly correlate with the duration of the disease; however, this study showed that swallowing function in the pharyngeal phase was not assessed fully by VF examination in MSA-C only. Combination with other instrumental evaluations, such as manometry and electromyography, may be useful, especially in the late stage of the disease. In addition, an analysis concerning the relationship between aspiration seen on VF examination and a history of aspiration pneumonia in MSA-C patients suggested that the sensory system at the larynx and trachea should also be assessed in patients in the late stage of MSA-C.

Silva et al. [71] evaluated three patients with MSA who showed impairment in the oral phase to solid food, with increased oral transit time and inefficient preparation of the bolus. In the pharyngeal phase, there was reduced laryngeal elevation and clinical signs of penetration and/or tracheal aspiration for solid and liquid consistencies. Postural maneuver (neck flexion) and cleaning of the pharyngeal recesses (swallowing effort and multiple swallows) were effective. The three patients had complaints in the oral phase of swallowing owing to motor changes already described in MSA; thus, the presence of dysarthria is an important signal in the differential diagnosis. The change in the pharyngeal phase of swallowing was mainly due to incoordination or reduced laryngeal elevation during the swallowing process. The subjects of this study benefited from postural maneuvers and cleaning the pharyngeal recesses, as the former increases airway protection and the latter helps to remove residues in pharyngeal recesses. Patients with MSA of this study showed oropharyngeal dysphagia with the same level of gravity. The speech therapy should be considered important in this disorder because patients described in this study showed improvement in swallowing.

Progressive Supranuclear Palsy

The dysphagia that occurs as an early sign of PSP, and which may predispose patients to aspiration pneumonia, has never been fully characterized. The study by Litvan et al. [72] evaluated 27 patients aged 64.9 years (mean age) with a symptom duration of 52 months who met the clinical National Institute of Neurological Disorders and Stroke and Society for PSP (NINDS-SPSP) criteria for possible or probable PSP, with a swallowing questionnaire, an oral motor and speech examination, and either a modified barium swallow or ultrasound study. Twenty-eight age- and sex-matched healthy controls aged 65.6 years (mean age) were also evaluated using the questionnaire, oral examination, and ultrasound study. Although PSP patients had at least one complaint on the swallowing questionnaire (mean, 6.6), healthy controls had fewer and less relevant complaints (0.3). Patients with moderate-to-severe cognitive disabilities had significantly more complaints of dysphagia than those with mild or no impairment. The oral motor skills and speech of the PSP patients were mildly impaired, but significantly different from those of controls. In the ultrasound studies, PSP patients had significantly fewer continuous swallows and required longer to complete their swallows than did healthy controls. They also had mild-to-moderate abnormalities in the modified barium swallow study. The swallowing questionnaire, oral motor examination, and speech production examination accurately predicted the abnormalities detected with the swallowing studies. Although 75% of patients had abnormal speech, all but one had abnormal swallowing studies. Thus, although dysphagia is associated with dysarthria, the two conditions are not always paired in the same patient. The authors suggest that the swallowing questionnaire and oral motor examination are an easy and cost-effective method for predicting the swallowing disturbances in PSP [72].

Corticobasal Syndrome

Ozsancak et al. [73] evaluated dysarthria and orofacial apraxia (OFA) in patients with a clinical diagnosis of CBS. Voluntary movements of the tongue and the lips were impaired in all patients. OFA, evaluated by simple and sequential gestures, was present in the patients. Sequential gestures were more frequently impaired. The OFA score did not correlate with the severity of dysarthria, suggesting independent underlying mechanisms. Thus, when specifically assessed, dysarthria and OFA are more frequent in CBS than usually reported. This study proposes that the underlying pathophysiology is the result of a deficit in programming and execution of repetitive movements.

Dysarthria is frequent in CBS even though it remains mild for a long period of time. The findings support the view that even though perceptual analysis is mandatory in the management of dysarthric patients, it does not help with the clinical differential diagnosis of CBS.

The study by Ozsancak et al. [74] suggests that the deficit in multiple sequential gestures in CBD might be related to simultaneous lesions of the parietal lobule and the supplementary motor area.

In a postmortem study, Müller et al. [56] confirmed that early dysarthria and perceived swallowing dysfunction are not features of PD. However, when one or both features were present, the sensitivity and specificity of their early occurrence within the first year failed to further distinguish among the various APDs. According to the findings of previous studies, dysarthria was frequently observed in all patients (MSD, PSP, CBS) [63, 75, 76], with significantly longer latencies in PD than in MSA and PSP. Similarly, dysarthria as a presenting symptom has been described in clinical series of CBS, MSA, and PSP [75]. In PD and DLB, hypophonic/monotonous speech represented the most frequent type of dysarthria, whereas imprecise or slurred articulation predominated in CBS, MSA, and PSP, in accordance with the literature [64, 75].

In a clinical study on CBS, Rinne et al. [75] described dysarthria as one of the initial symptoms in 11 % of the patients. At follow-up, on average 5.2 years, dysarthria was diagnosed in 70 % of the patients. In a study of 147 CBS cases, including 7 autopsy-confirmed CBD cases, dysarthria was noted only in 29 % of patients, but there was no information on disease duration [77]. According to the findings of Müller et al. [56], dysarthria occurred in almost every patient with CBS/CBD.

Median latencies to dysarthria and subjective dysphagia were at least twice as long in PD than in APDs. Total survival time, in addition to survival time after onset of dysarthria, was significantly longer in PD; however, the onset of dysphagia predicted a similarly short remaining median survival time in MSA, PSP, and PD. Furthermore, latencies to dysphagia correlated highly with overall survival time in all parkinsonian disorders. These important findings suggest that the perceived swallowing dysfunction in PD and APDs might indicate functionally relevant dysphagia. Indeed, in PD [77], DLB [78], CBS [79], MSA [80], and PSP [72], bronchopneumonia has been reported to be a leading cause of death, which may be subsequent to silent aspiration resulting from dysphagia. Thus, evaluation and adequate treatment of parkinsonian patients who complain of dysphagia may prevent or delay complications such as aspiration pneumonia and increase survival time in these patients. Also, an appropriate and timely swallowing evaluation may provide patients and caregivers with techniques and resources that may in turn improve their quality of life (e.g., straws, food thickeners, and percutaneous endoscopic gastrostomy). Patients with MSA and PSP complained of a swallowing dysfunction, in contrast to patients with PD, CBS, and DLB. In PD, the reported prevalence of dysphagia varies from 18.5 to 100 % [80], depending on the measurement method. Investigators who carried out assessment with barium swallow found abnormalities in all study patients with PD [81], and complaints of dysphagia in patients with PD were found to correlate poorly with radiological and videofluoroscopic findings [81]. Impaired lingual proprioception is hypothesized to contribute to the unawareness of swallowing difficulties in PD and may partly explain significantly longer latencies to dysphagia in our PD cases. In contrast, patients with PSP were reported to be keenly aware of swallowing problems, including those with cognitive impairment [72]. In a clinical study on swallowing abnormalities in PSP, Litvan et al. [72] reported abnormal results on modified barium swallow or ultrasound studies in 96 % of patients, which exceeds the 83 % dysphagia in our PSP cases, a finding that is probably related to the higher sensitivity of objective measurements. However, the similarly short remaining survival time in PD and PSP after the onset of perceived dysphagia suggests that this symptom might represent a reliable marker for the onset of functionally relevant swallowing abnormalities in both disorders. Similar to PSP, dysphagia within the first year of disease onset was observed in MSA, and dysphagia was a frequent complaint in MSA.

In CBS, dysphagia was noticed in 31 % of cases after a median disease duration of 64 months in the study by Müller et al. [56]. Dysphagia in CBS is believed to result from bulbar dysfunction, which is uncommon initially, but often appears after several years of disease [82]. Accordingly, none of patients with CBS noticed early dysphagia. To our knowledge, dysphagia has not yet been investigated systematically in CBS, and the two largest studies, by Kompoliti et al. [77] (147 cases) and Rinne et al. [75] (36 cases), provided no data on the frequency or latency of dysphagia.

The findings of increased latency to dysarthria and dysphagia and a similar time interval from onset of dysphagia to death in patients with PD compared with patients with APDs suggest that extra-striatal and nondopaminergic lesions might represent an important factor in the development of dysarthria and dysphagia. Whereas the APDs are characterized by multiple system neuronal degenerations, in PD disease progression is determined by a progressive dopaminergic deficit arising from the selective neuronal degeneration of the pars compacta of the substantia nigra. It may be the overall degenerative lesion load in excess of the dopaminergic projection that shortens the onset of axial features, such as dysarthria and dysphagia, and therefore predicts poor survival in patients with PD. However, the presence of distinct neuropathological lesion patterns in these disorders suggests that disease-specific factors might contribute to the pathophysiological processes underlying dysarthria and dysphagia.

In relation to swallowing changes in the advanced phases of APDs, patients may have a lack of laryngeal closure during swallowing and consequently aspiration, because as described above, penetration was observed, with sequential aspiration. Consequently, swallowing disorders could be associated with considerable morbidity, under-nutrition, lack of hydration, and pulmonary sequelae [83]. However, patients are usually referred for or seek hearing assistance when complaints present and the symptoms are already at a more advanced stage; when, for example, choking is common during meals, or it becomes necessary to reduce the consistency and quantity of food, leading the patient to a state of debilitation, in extreme cases requiring the use of a nasogastric or gastrostomy tube. When dysphagia is detected early, the patient can practically resume normal deglutition and even delay the evolution of this change, in view of the progressive aspect of the disease.

This is possibly due to muscle rigidity, bradykinesia, or even akinesia and a lack of coordination of movements present in the disease, inducing weakness and incapacity of the oral muscles. At the loss of these muscles, the food is not well masticated and eating may result in coughing and/or gagging, or more frequently throat clearing.

In the advanced stage of APDs, we observed clinically frequent impairment in patients in swallowing his/her own saliva, or the automatic engine movement is no longer performed, inducing an excessive amount of saliva in the oral cavity, which may then escape through the lips, making it a compelling factor in the social environment or disrupting the correct emission of speech sounds, compromising intelligibility, or when the saliva accumulates in the pharynx, and not swallowed, the possibility of gagging also increases and gives the distressing sensation of a wet voice, which makes it difficult to understand speech. Furthermore, the presence of large amounts of saliva can hinder the performance of exercises during the speech therapy of voice, speech, and/or deglutition.

References

1. Mark MH. Lumping and splitting the Parkinson plus syndromes: dementia with Lewy bodies, multiple system atrophy, progressive supranuclear palsy, and cortico-basal ganglionic degeneration. Neurol Clin. 2001;19:607–27.
2. Stamelou M, Bhatia KP. Atypical parkinsonism. Diagnosis and treatment. Neurol Clin. 2015;33(1):39–56.
3. Siuda J, Fujioka S, Wszolek ZK. Parkinsonian syndrome in familial frontotemporal dementia. Parkinsonism Relat Disord. 2014;20(9):957–64.
4. Wenning GK, Ben-Shlomo Y, Magalhães M, et al. Clinicopathological study of 35 cases of multiple system atrophy. J Neurol Neurosurg Psychiatry. 1995;58:160–6.
5. Schrag A, Ben-Shlomo Y, Quinn NP. Prevalence of progressive supranuclear palsy and multiple system atrophy: a cross-sectional study. Lancet. 1999;354:1771–5.
6. Stefanova N, Bucke P, Duerr S, Wenning GK. Multiple system atrophy: an update. Lancet Neurol. 2009;8:1172–8.
7. Gilman S, Low PA, Quinn N, et al. Consensus statement on the diagnosis of multiple system atrophy. J Neurol Sci. 1999;163:94–8.
8. Ahmed Z, Asi YT, Sailer A, Lees AJ, Houlden H, Revesz T, Holton JL. The neuropathology, pathophysiology and genetics of multiple system atrophy. Neuropathol Appl Neurobiol. 2012;38(1):4–24.

9. Multiple-System Atrophy Research Collaboration. Mutations in COQ2 in familial and sporadic multiple-system atrophy. N Engl J Med. 2013;369(3):233–44.
10. Bhattacharya K, Saadia D, Eisenkraft B, et al. Brain magnetic resonance imaging in multiple system atrophy and Parkinson disease: a diagnostic algorithm. Arch Neurol. 2002;59:835–42.
11. Dodel R, Spottke A, Gerhard A, Reuss A, Reinecker S, et al. Minocycline 1-year therapy in multiple-system-atrophy: effect on clinical symptoms and [(11)C] (R)-PK11195 PET (MEMSA-trial). Mov Disord. 2010;25(1):97–107.
12. Poewe W, Mahlknecht P, Krismer F. Therapeutic advances in multiple system atrophy and progressive supranuclear palsy. Mov Disord. 2015;30(11):1528–38.
13. Steele JC, Richardson JC, Progressive OJ, Palsy S. A heterogeneous degeneration involving the brain stem, basal ganglia and cerebellum with vertical gaze and pseudobulbar palsy, nuchal dystonia and dementia. Arch Neurol. 1964;10:333–59.
14. Santacruz P, Uttl B, Litvan I, Grafman J. Progressive supranuclear palsy: a survey of the disease course. Neurology. 1998;50:1637–47.
15. Barsottini OG, Felício AC, Aquino CC, Pedroso JL. Progressive supranuclear palsy: new concepts. Arq Neuropsiquiatr. 2010;68(6):938–46.
16. Lopez G, Bayulkem K, Hallett M. Progressive supranuclear palsy (PSP): Richardson syndrome and other PSP variants. Acta Neurol Scand. 2016. doi:10.1111/ane.12546.
17. Ling H. Clinical approach to progressive supranuclear palsy. J Mov Disord. 2016;9(1):3–13.
18. Litvan I, Agid Y, Calne D, Campbell G, Dubois B, et al. Clinical research criteria for the diagnosis of progressive supranuclear palsy (Steele-Richardson-Olszewski syndrome): report of the NINDS-SPSP international workshop. Neurology. 1996;47(1):1–9.
19. Kanazawa M, Shimohata T, Toyoshima Y, Tada M, Kakita A, Morita T, Ozawa T, Takahashi H, Nishizawa M. Cerebellar involvement in progressive supranuclear palsy: a clinicopathological study. Mov Disord. 2009;24(9):1312–18.
20. Barsottini OG, Ferraz HB, Maia Jr AC, Silva CJ, Rocha AJ. Differentiation of Parkinson's disease and progressive supranuclear palsy with magnetic resonance imaging: the first Brazilian experience. Parkinsonism Relat Disord. 2007;13(7):389–93.
21. Rebeiz J, Kolodny E, Richardson E. Corticodentatonigral degeneration with neuronal achromasia: a progressive disorder of late adult life. Trans Am Neurol Assoc. 1967;92:23–6.
22. Armstrong MJ, Litvan I, Lang AE, Bak TH, Bhatia KP, et al. Criteria for the diagnosis of corticobasal degeneration. Neurology. 2013;80(5):496–503.
23. Wadia PM, Lang AE. The many faces of corticobasal degeneration. Parkinsonism Relat Disord. 2007;3:S336–40.
24. Grijalvo-Perez AM, Litvan I. Corticobasal degeneration. Semin Neurol. 2014;34(2):160–73.
25. Stamelou M, Quinn NP, Bhatia KP. "Atypical" Atypical parkinsonism (APD): new genetic conditions presenting with features of progressive supranuclear palsy, corticobasal degeneration, or multiple system atrophy-a diagnostic guide. Mov Disord. 2013;28(9):1184–99.
26. Seppi K, Poewe W. Brain magnetic resonance imaging techniques in the diagnosis of parkinsonian syndromes. Neuroimaging Clin N Am. 2010;20(1):29–55.
27. Nonnekes J, Aerts MB, Abdo WF, Bloem B. Medio-lateral balance impairment differentiates between Parkinson disease and atypical parkinsonism. J Parkinsons Dis. 2014;4:567–9.
28. Abdo WF, Borm GF, Munneke M, Verbeek MM, Esselink RA, Bloem BR. Ten steps to identify atypical parkinsonism. J Neurol Neurosurg Psychiatry. 2006;77:1367–9.
29. Aerts MB, Abdo WF, Bloem BR. The "bicycle sign" for atypical parkinsonism. Lancet. 2011;377:125–6.
30. Suteerawattananon M, MacNeill B, Protas EJ. Supported treadmill training for gait and balance in a patient with progressive supranuclear palsy. Phys Ther. 2002;82:485–95.
31. Steffen TM, Boeve BF, Mollinger-Riemann LA, Petersen CM. Long-term locomotor training for gait and balance in a patient with mixed progressive supranuclear palsy and corticobasal degeneration. Phys Ther. 2007;87:1078–108.
32. Steffen TM, Boeve BF, Kantarci K. Long-term exercise training for an individual with mixed corticobasal degeneration and progressive supranuclear palsy features: 10-year case report follow-up. Phys Ther. 2014;94(2):289–96.

33. Hollands MA, Patla AE, Vickers JN. "Look where you're going!": gaze behaviour associated with maintaining and changing the direction of locomotion. Exp Brain Res. 2002;143:221–30.
34. Di Fabio RP, Greany J, Zampieri C. Saccade-stepping interactions revise the motor plan for obstacle avoidance. J Mot Behav. 2003;35:383–97.
35. Di Fabio RP, Zampieri C, Henke J, Olsen K, Rickheim D, Russell M. Influence of elderly executive cognitive function on attention in the lower visual field during step initiation. Gerontology. 2005;51:94–107.
36. Lindemann U, Nicolai S, Beische D, et al. Clinical and dual-tasking aspects in frequent and infrequent fallers with progressive supranuclear palsy. Mov Disord. 2010;25:1040–6.
37. Zampieri C, Di Fabio RP. Improvement of gaze control after balance and eye movement training in patients with progressive supranuclear palsy: a quasi-randomized controlled trial. Arch Phys Med Rehabil. 2009;90:263–70.
38. Seamon B, DeFranco M, Thigpen M. Use of the Xbox kinect virtual gaming system to improve gait, postural control and cognitive awareness in an individual with progressive supranuclear palsy. Disabil Rehabil. 2016;23:1–6.
39. Tison F, Yekhlef F, Chrysostome V, Balestre E, Quinn NP, Poewe W, Wenning GK. Parkinsonism in multiple system atrophy: natural history, severity (UPDRS-III), and disability assessment compared with Parkinson's disease. Mov Disord. 2002;17:701–9.
40. Van De Warrenburg BP, Cordivari C, Ryan AM, Phadke R, Holton JL, Bhatia KP, Hanna MG, Quinn NP. The phenomenon of disproportionate antecollis in Parkinson's disease and multiple system atrophy. Mov Disord. 2007;22:2325–31.
41. Wedge F. The impact of resistance training on balance and functional ability of a patient with multiple system atrophy. J Geriatr Phys Ther. 2008;31:79–83.
42. Liu T, Lao L. Tai chi for patients with Parkinson's disease. N Engl J Med. 2012;3:1737–40.
43. Schroeteler FE. Tai Chi Chuan improves balance and gait in people with Parkinson's disease. MMW Fortschr Med. 2013;8:52–3.
44. Yang Y, Qiu WQ, Hao YL, Lv ZY, Jiao SJ, Teng JF. The efficacy of traditional Chinese medical exercise for Parkinson's disease: a systematic review and meta-analysis. PLoS One. 2015;4:1–10.
45. Venglar M. Case report: Tai Chi and parkinsonism. Physiother Res Int. 2005;10:116–21.
46. Batista CS, Kanegusuku H, Roschel H, Souza EO, Cunha TF, Laurentino GC, Junior MN, De Mello MT, Piemonte MEP, Brum PC, Forjaz CL, Tricoli V, Ugrinowitsch C. Resistance training with instability in multiple system atrophy: a case report. J Sports Sci Med. 2014;13:597–603.
47. Freeman R. Clinical practice. Neurogenic orthostatic hypotension. N Engl J Med. 2008;358(6):615–24.
48. Ooi WL, Hossain M, Lipsitz LA. The association between orthostatic hypotension and recurrent falls in nursing home residents. Am J Med. 2000;108(2):106–11.
49. Low PA, Opfer-Gehrking TL, McPhee BR, et al. Prospective evaluation of clinical characteristics of orthostatic hypotension. Mayo Clin Proc. 1995;70(7):617–22.
50. Milazzo V, Di Stefano C, Servo S, et al. Drugs and orthostatic hypotension: evidence from literature. J Hypertens. 2012;1(2):1–8.
51. Mills PB, Fung CK, Travlos A, Krassioukov A. Nonpharmacologic management of orthostatic hypotension: a systematic review. Arch Phys Med Rehabil. 2015;96(2):366–75.
52. Shibao C, Lipsitz LA, Biaggioni I. Evaluation and treatment of orthostatic hypotension. J Am Soc Hypertens. 2013;7:317–24.
53. Isaacson SH, Skettini J. Neurogenic orthostatic hypotension in Parkinson's disease: evaluation, management, and emerging role of droxidopa. Vasc Health Risk Manag. 2014;10:169–76.
54. Kawahira K, Noma T, Iiyama J, Etoh S, Ogata A, Shimodozono M. Improvements in limb kinetic apraxia by repetition of a newly designed facilitation exercise in a patient with corticobasal degeneration. Int J Rehabil Res. 2009;32(2):178–83.
55. Shehata HS, Shalaby NM, Esmail EH, Fahmy E. Corticobasal degeneration: clinical characteristics and multidisciplinary therapeutic approach in 26 patients. Neurol Sci. 2015;36(9):1651–7.

56. Müller J, Wenning GK, Verny M, McKee A, Chaudhuri KR, Jellinger K, Poewe W, Litvan I. Progression of dysarthria and dysphagia in postmortem-confirmed parkinsonian disorders. Arch Neurol. 2001;58(2):259–64. doi:10.1001/archneur.58.2.259.

57. International Medical Workshop. Covering progressive supranuclear palsy, multiple system atrophy, and cortico basal degeneration. Mov Disord. 2001;16:382–95.

58. Siemers E. Multiple system atrophy. Med Clin N Am. 1999;83:381–92.

59. Darley FL, Aronson A, Brown JR. Differential diagnostic patterns of dysarthria. J Speech Hear Res. 1969;12:246–52.

60. Darley FL, Aronson A, Brown JR. Clusters of deviant speech dimensions in disarthrias. J Speech Hear Res. 1969;12:462–8.

61. Knopp D, Barsottini OGP, Ferraz HB. Avaliação fonoaudiológica na atrofia de múltiplos sistemas: estudo com cinco pacientes. Arq Neuro-Psiquiatr. 2002;60:3A.

62. Countryman S, Ramig LO, Pawlas AA. Speech and voice deficits in parkinsonian plus syndromes: can they be treated? J Med Speech Lang Pathol. 1994;2:211–25.

63. Wenning GK, Ben Shlomo Y, Magalhães M, Daniel SE, Quinn NP. Clinical features and natural history of multiple system atrophy. Brain. 1994;117:835–45.

64. Quinn N. Multiple system atrophy: the nature of the beast. J Neurol Neurosurg Psychiatry. 1989;52:78–89.

65. De Angelis EC. Deglutição, configuração laríngea, análise clínica e acústica computadorizada da voz de pacientes com doença de Parkinson. São Paulo: Tese de Doutorado, Universidade Federal de São Paulo; 2000.

66. Duffy JR. Motor speech disorders: substrates, differential diagnosis and management. St. Louis: Mosby; 1995.

67. Hanson DG, Ludlow CL, Bassich CJ. Vocal fold paresis in Shy-Drager syndrome. Ann Otol Rhinol Laryngol. 1983;92:85–90.

68. Kluin KJ, Gilman S, Lohman M, Junck L. Characteristics of the dysarthria of multiple system atrophy. Arch Neurol. 1996;53:545–8.

69. Rehman HU. Multiple system atrophy. Postgrad Med J. 2001;77:379–82.

70. Higo R, Nito T, Tayama N. Swallowing function in patients with multiple-system atrophy with a clinical predominance of cerebellar symptoms (MSA-C). Eur Arch Otorhinolaryngol. 2005;262(8):646–50.

71. Silva AB, Chiari BM, Lima CF, Gonçalves MIR, Lira M, Souza NC. A deglutição na atrofia de múltiplos sistemas—estudo com três pacientes. In: Anais do 19° congresso brasileiro e 8° congresso internacional de fonoaudiologia. 30 de outubro a 02 de novembro de 2011; São Paulo, Brasil. São Paulo: Sociedade Brasileira de Fonoaudiologia; 2011.

72. Litvan I, Sastry N, Sonies BC. Characterizing swallowing abnormalities in progressive supranuclear palsy. Neurology. 1997;48(6):1654–62.

73. Ozsancak C, Auzou P, Hannequin D. Dysarthria and orofacial apraxia in corticobasal degeneration. Mov Disord. 2000;15(5):905–10.

74. Ozsancak C, Auzou P, Jan M, Defebvre L, Derambure P, Destee A. The place of perceptual analysis of dysarthria in the differential diagnosis of corticobasal degeneration and Parkinson's disease. J Neurol. 2006;253(1):92–7.

75. Rinne JO, Lee MS, Thompson PD, Marsden CD. Corticobasal degeneration: a clinical study of 36 cases. Brain. 1994;117:1183–96.

76. Johnston BT, Castell JA, Stumacher S, et al. Comparison of swallowing function in Parkinson's disease and progressive supranuclear palsy. Mov Disord. 1997;12:322–7.

77. Kompoliti K, Goetz CG, Boeve BF, et al. Clinical presentation and pharmacological therapy in corticobasal degeneration. Arch Neurol. 1998;55:957–61.

78. Hely MA, Reid WGJ, Halliday GM, et al. Diffuse Lewy body disease: clinical features in nine cases without coexistent Alzheimer's disease. J Neurol Neurosurg Psychiatry. 1996;60:531–8.

79. Wenning GK, Litvan I, Jankovic J, et al. Natural history and survival of 14 patients with corticobasal degeneration confirmed at postmortem examination. J Neurol Neurosurg Psychiatry. 1998;64:184–9.

80. Wenning GK, Tison F, Ben Shlomo Y, Daniel SE, Quinn NP. Multiple system atrophy: a review of 203 pathologically proven cases. Mov Disord. 1997;12:133–47.
81. Robbins JA, Logemann JA, Kirshner HS. Swallowing and speech production in Parkinson's disease. Ann Neurol. 1986;19:283–7.
82. Kumar R, Bergeron C, Pollanen MS, Lang AE. Cortical-basal ganglionic degeneration. In: Jankovic J, Tolosa E, editors. Parkinson's disease and movement disorders. Baltimore, MD: Williams & Wilkins; 1998. p. 297–316.
83. Lieberman AN, Horowitz L, Redmond P, Pachter L, Lieber-mann I, Leibowitz M. Dysphagia in Parkinson's disease. Am J Gastroenterol. 1980;74:157–60.

Rehabilitation of Dystonia

4

Dirk Dressler and Fereshte Adib Saberi

Introduction

Dystonia is a syndrome describing a special form of muscle hyperactivity characterised by "sustained or intermittent muscle contractions causing abnormal, often repetitive movements, postures, or both. Dystonic movements are typically patterned, twisting, and may be tremulous. Dystonia is often initiated or worsened by voluntary action and associated with overflow muscle activation" [1]. Dystonic muscle hyperactivity is often painful and may produce complications in connective tissues, ligaments, the spinal cord, nerve roots, peripheral nerves, blood vessels, spinal discs and joints.

Dystonia is usually classified according to its location within the body. Cranial dystonia includes periocular dystonia (blepharospasm), mandibular dystonia, perioral dystonia, lingual dystonia and combinations of these (oromandibular dystonia, Meige syndrome: blepharospasm and other forms of cranial dystonia). Cervical dystonia may be distinguished according to the patient's predominant head postures. Distinguishing between deviations of the head and those of the neck, numerous postures may be described: torticollis, laterocollis, laterocaput, antecollis, antecaput, retrocollis, retrocaput, anterior sagittal shift (antecollis and retrocaput), posterior sagittal shift (retrocollis and antecaput), lateral shift (laterocollis and contralateral laterocaput). Dystonia may also be localised to the pharynx, larynx (spasmodic dysphonia), in limbs and in axial muscles. In focal dystonia one body region is affected; the terms segmental, multisegmental and generalised dystonia describe more wide-spread involvement. Other classifications are based on the age at manifestation, the continuity of occurrence (continuous,

D. Dressler, M.D., Ph.D. (✉) • F. Adib Saberi, M.D.
Movement Disorders Section, Department of Neurology, Hannover Medical School, Hannover, Germany
e-mail: dressler.dirk@mh-hannover.de

© Springer International Publishing Switzerland 2017
H.F. Chien, O.G.P. Barsottini (eds.), *Movement Disorders Rehabilitation*, DOI 10.1007/978-3-319-46062-8_4

intermittent, paroxysmal) and the conditions of occurrence (task-specific, action-induced, spontaneous). Causal factors may also be considered for classification: idiopathic, symptomatic owing to structural lesions, pharmacological interactions, metabolic disorders and psychogenic reactions. In idiopathic dystonia a genetic predisposition and epigenetic triggering factors are assumed. Triggering factors may be extreme stress, functional overuse and age. Dystonia may occur as an isolated symptom or in the context of other symptoms or conditions. The prototypical dystonia patient suffers from idiopathic cervical dystonia or blepharospasm starting in his sixth or seventh decade of life, showing slow progression over a few years and then reaching a stationary course.

Pathophysiology includes a lack of cortical inhibition arising from basal ganglia dysfunction. Genetic predisposition seems likely; however, an extremely low penetrance indicates the major importance of epigenetic factors that are, however, largely unidentified.

Depending on the location of the dystonia differential diagnoses include tics, hemifacial spasm, tremor, myoclonus, myasthenia gravis, ptosis, eyelid dehiscence, focal polymyositis, dens subluxation, traumatic torticollis, ocular or vestibular torticollis. Diagnosis of dystonia is focussed on identification of treatable courses such as tumours, infections, dopa responsiveness and rare metabolic conditions such as Wilson's disease. In prototypical cases the diagnostic process is brief and straightforward; however, in atypical cases complex metabolic and genetic testing may become necessary.

The overall frequency of dystonia is difficult to describe, as the severity varies greatly. It is probably half that the frequency of parkinsonism. In declining order, the relative frequency is cervical dystonia, blepharospasm, writer's cramp, laryngeal dystonia (spasmodic dysphonia), segmental/multisegmental dystonia and generalised dystonia.

The course of dystonia is chronic, with slow progression during the first years and a plateau phase thereafter. It is important to realise for the patient and the physician that dystonia is not continuously progressive like other neurodegenerative disorders. Equally important for the patient is the fact that idiopathic dystonia does not affect cognitive function in a clinically relevant way.

Special Features of Dystonia

Dystonia has a number of special features that are relevant to therapeutic interventions. It can be substantially modified by a number of factors (Table 4.1), one of which is psychological tension. Psychological stress and anxiety usually aggravate dystonia, whereas relaxation improves it. Another modifying factor is changing the sensory input to the central nervous system either on somatosensory or proprioceptive pathways. Wearing silk scarves may reduce cervical dystonia and changing the texture of the pen may reduce writer's cramp. Changing the

Table 4.1 Modifiers of dystonia

Modifier		Dystonia type affected	Effect on dystonia
Tension	Stress, anxiety	All	↑
	Relaxation	All	↓
Sensory input	Wearing silk scarves	CD	↓
	Changing the texture of the pen	WC	↓
Motor output	General motor activation (overflow)	All	↑
	Forced postures	All	↑
	Dancing, horse riding	All	↓
	Using print characters	WC	↓
	Changing the position of the pen and the arm	WC	↓
	Changing the position of the musical instrument	MC	↓
	Singing, increasing the pitch	SD	↓
Sensory input and	Geste antagoniste	CD	↓
	Touching the lateral periocular skin	BS	↓
Motor output	Biting matches, using chewing gum	OMD	↓

BS blepharospasm, *CD* cervical dystonia, *OMD* oromandibular dystonia, *MC* musician's cramp, *WC* writer's cramp

motor activity of the central nervous system may also be a modifying factor of dystonia. General physical activity and forced postures usually increase dystonia (overflow effect), whereas resting and relaxation improve it. When negative physical activity is combined with psychological tension, as is the case when working on a production line without being able to interrupt the mechanics, the effect may be disastrous. On the other hand, working at a self-paced speed with self-set pauses and a change of position is often a relief for the patient. Rhythmic activities such as dancing and horse-riding may improve all forms of dystonia. When using print characters, changing the position of the pen and the arm may improve writer's cramp, changing the position of the musical instrument may be beneficial for musician's cramps, and singing and increasing the pitch may improve spasmodic dysphonia. Changing dystonically impaired motor programmes can be effective. This approach is frequently used in occupational therapy re-training programmes, especially in task-specific dystonia. Amending both the motor output from the central nervous system and the sensory input to the central nervous system may produce very specific effects. The geste antagoniste, the combination of a self-intended movement or posture and the elucidation of sensory effects in the patient, reduces cervical dystonia and dystonic neck tremor. It is specific to dystonia and is not seen in other conditions. Effects on the "wrong" side of the chin indicate that the geste antagoniste is not a mechanical manoeuvre. Imitation of the sensory effect via an external source is not effective. Touching the lateral periocular skin, a sensory manoeuvre similar to the geste antagoniste, may reduce blepharospasm; biting matches and using chewing gum may lessen oromandibular dystonia.

Treatment of Dystonia

Dystonia is a chronic condition. In idiopathic dystonia, by far the most common form of dystonia, the cause is not known and in symptomatic dystonia most causes are not reversible. The typical treatment of dystonia, therefore, has to be symptomatic and long-term [2]. As no single treatment option produces complete remission of the symptoms, combinations of different treatment modalities often become necessary. Disease-modifying treatments are not known.

Antidystonic Treatment

Botulinum toxin (BT) therapy is the most effective way of relaxing dystonic muscle hyperactivity. BT produces a strictly local, well controllable and fully reversible blockade of the cholinergic neuromuscular synapse for approximately 3 months. Its application is based upon an injection scheme including the target muscles and their BT doses. The development of appropriate injection schemes greatly depends on the experience of the injector. Most cases of "therapy failure" are actually caused by inappropriate injection schemes and are therefore "therapist failure". Best results are obtained in focal dystonia. However, recent publications indicate that total BT doses are higher than previously thought; thus, more widespread dystonia can also be targeted [3]. Dystonic muscle activity can also be suppressed by *surgical interventions*. Deep brain stimulation (DBS) blocks certain basal ganglia pathways by continuous high frequency stimulation through stereotactically implanted electrodes. Target of the stimulation is the globus pallidus internus. For tremor-type dystonia thalamic targets may also be used. DBS works best in idiopathic dystonia. It has a far-reaching effect and is therefore recommended for non-focal dystonia. A combination of posterior ramisectomy, peripheral denervation and myectomy of the sternocleidomastoid muscle is called the Bertrand procedure [3]. Before BT therapy it was commonly used with some success to treat cervical dystonia. Other selective denervations and myectomies may be used in special forms of very localised dystonia. Spinal cord stimulation turned out not to be effective.

Antidystonic Drugs

A large number of drugs were tried to treat dystonia. In general, drug treatment of dystonia is disappointing as it is usually ineffective and often accompanied by severe adverse effects. Best antidystonic effects are produced by anticholinergic drugs, especially in children tolerating high doses. Antidopaminergic drugs may also be helpful. Dopamine receptor blocking agents, however, bear the risk of inducing tardive dystonia; dopamine-depleting agents do not, but often produce parkinsonism and depression. GABA-ergic compounds have also documented antidystonic efficacy. Continuous intrathecal baclofen administered through an implanted pump was tried with mixed results in non-focal dystonia [5].

Adjuvant Drugs

Analgesics may be used if there are painful secondary complications and when the painful dystonic muscle activity cannot be sufficiently suppressed otherwise. Anxiolytics can reduce stress as a dystonia facilitating factor. Knowing that there is the option to use them sometimes helps.

Rehabilitation of Dystonia

Methods

Rehabilitation of dystonia includes a number of therapeutic interventions such as physiotherapy, occupational therapy, speech therapy, psychotherapy and the use of orthoses. Additionally, counselling of the patient and his/her family plays an important role. The goals of rehabilitation of dystonia include re-training of normal postures and movement patterns, prevention and therapy of secondary complications and coping with pain and the burden of a chronic disease.

Structural Aspects

As dystonia is a chronic condition and there is no cure for it, rehabilitation of dystonia needs to be provided continuously. The combination of methods applied and their frequency and intensity depend on the severity of the patient's individual dystonia. It is best offered on an outpatient basis within the patient's community. This concept of rehabilitation of dystonia, however, does not match the traditional concept of rehabilitation as a short intense inpatient intervention to correct an acute deficit. Structures to provide appropriate rehabilitation of dystonia are lacking in many health care systems. One strategy to overcome this deficit is the Interdisciplinary Working Group for Movement Disorders (IAB) [6]. It is a network of medical and non-medical and inpatient and outpatient movement disorder therapists dedicated to interdisciplinary collaboration. It is based on regional groups backed up by a central office providing various data bases, educational material and scores and scales to harmonise the evaluation of movement disorders and their therapies. Recently, the IAB started the IAB Academy, providing government-accredited, structuralised education for movement disorder specialists.

Another problem of rehabilitation of dystonia is the lack of academic and scientific structures in many countries. Compared with other health care sectors the disease terminology and the descriptions of interventions are often ambiguous. Coupled with a general lack of robust studies, it is therefore difficult to compare and evaluate the efficacy of the rehabilitative interventions offered [7].

Cervical Dystonia

Figure 4.1 shows some typical patients with cervical dystonia. BT therapy is the treatment of choice for cervical dystonia. In patients with special forms of dystonia, such as antecollis, antecaput, tremor forms or alternating forms, and in patients with antibody-induced therapy failure, DBS is an alternative. Antidystonic drugs and adjuvant drugs may be used at the end of the BT treatment cycle. When BT therapy is used, physiotherapy is necessary in most patients to activate antidystonic muscles and to re-learn the normal head position. It also helps to mobilise existing contractures or to prevent them. Based on these principles and on several decades of

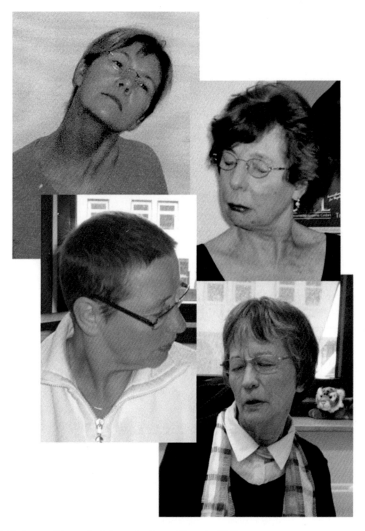

Fig. 4.1 Patients with cervical dystonia. From: Dressler [74]

practical experience, Bleton has developed a physiotherapeutic training programme [8] that is now used in many countries around the world. However, a recent study challenged its efficacy [8]. Other studies demonstrated that physiotherapy may reduce BT doses [10, 11].

Behavioural therapy is mainly based on electromyographic feedback techniques. Nine studies used feedback techniques with some success and sometimes continued improvement [12–19]. However, only two of them [14, 16] used a randomised design. Other behavioural techniques [20–22] are based on changes in the sensory input to the central nervous system [23, 24]. Vestibular stimulation [25] and orthosis [25] were occasionally used in small case series with mixed results.

Blepharospasm

Figure 4.2 shows some typical patients with blepharospasm and Meige syndrome. The treatment of choice for blepharospasm is BT therapy. It produces robust improvement in most patients treated. In some patients, results are less favourable, usually because of additional eyelid opening apraxia (levator inhibition) preventing appropriate activation of the levator palpebrae muscle. Levator suspension operation [27] connecting the upper eyelid to the frontalis muscle via a Goretex® string is helpful. Alternatively, a spring attached to a spectacle's frame may help (Fig. 4.3). Patients starting to use plasters usually report skin irritations after a short period of time. DBS

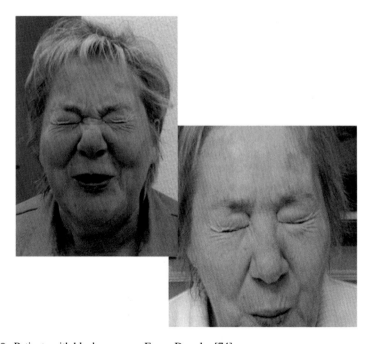

Fig. 4.2   Patients with blepharospasm. From: Dressler [74]

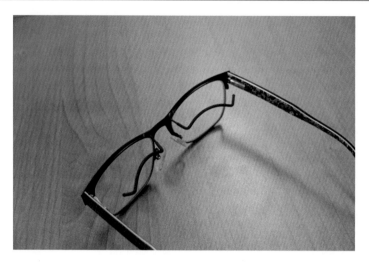

Fig. 4.3 Springs attached to a spectacles frame to cope with eyelid opening apraxia as part of blepharospasm

is principally effective in blepharospasm; however, BT therapy is considerably less invasive. Peripheral denervation operations are obsolete because of frequent excessive periorbital pain and uncontrollable effects.

Rehabilitation of blepharospasm is mainly based on electromyographic feedback strategies developed in the 1970s [28–33]. Reducing factors facilitating the normal blink reflex, such as bright light and cold air by wearing sunglasses may be helpful.

Laryngeal and Pharyngeal Dystonia

Laryngeal dystonia (spasmodic dysphonia) is an extremely rewarding indication for BT therapy. Adductor as well as abductor forms respond well. BT may be applied transcutaneously under electromyographic monitoring or transorally under direct visual control. Pharyngeal dystonia often occurring in patients with tardive dystonia may also be treated with BT therapy.

Rehabilitation of spasmodic dysphonia is usually applied as speech therapy. Speech therapy tries to improve breathing, tongue, lip and mandibular movements and tries to maintain a dystonia-free phonation. The basic idea is to focus attention on these single elements and to train for optimal performance. General recommendations include avoidance of stress, of voice overuse and of unfavourable situations, including talking over the phone and noisy places.

Blitzer and colleagues [35] found in a retrospective review of 110 patients with spasmodic dysphonia that speech therapy, psychotherapy and feedback techniques had limited success, whereas one third of patients benefited from systemic medication and all patients improved with BT therapy. Speech therapy may increase the duration of BT therapy in spasmodic dysphonia [35].

Rehabilitation of pharyngeal dystonia is usually aimed at improving swallowing. It is usually applied by speech therapists as swallowing therapy. Again, it is based on focusing attention on the single elements of the swallowing process and on training their optimised performance. General recommendations include changing the food consistency to either liquid or solid, careful food preparation, thorough chewing, eating under optimal conditions (no distraction, upright body position) and repeated clearing of the throat. Nasogastric tube feeding will only rarely become necessary and should be avoided if possible.

Task-Specific Dystonia

Figure 4.4 shows some typical patients with task-specific dystonia. For writer's cramp and musician's cramps, the most common forms of task-specific dystonia, BT is the treatment of choice. However, for writer's cramp one third to half of the patients are not satisfied with BT therapy. For musician's cramps, with their excessive functional demands, this percentage is higher. Oral antidystonic drugs are problematic owing to weak and unpredictable effects and potentially severe adverse effects. In musician's cramps, however, trihexyphenidyl is frequently used [36]. Adjuvant drugs, especially anxiolytics, may be additionally helpful. DBS was tried in single cases with mixed results. In this situation, rehabilitation is in high demand, especially in patients with musician's dystonia when their ability to perform professionally is at stake.

Originally, it was thought that task-specific dystonia was a functional disorder, a software problem triggered by overuse. Although overuse, especially under stressful circumstances, seems to play a major role in the pathophysiology of task-specific dystonia, it has become increasingly apparent that the pathological basis of task-specific dystonia is not principally different from that of other forms of dystonia. Still, the strong correlation with special motor programmes is intriguing and has stimulated treatment with movement-modifying programmes.

Over many years of practical work with writer's cramp patients, Bleton developed a physiotherapy programme based on the concept of re-learning normal movements by improving independence and the precision of individual finger and wrist movements and training of antidystonic muscles by drawing loops, curves and arabesques [37]. Occupational therapy is even more widely used and employs a large number of different strategies, including simple ones such as switching writing hands, writing in print, using keyboards and—where possible—speech recognition devices, changing to thick pens and pens with a non-slippery surface, altering the pen-holding position [38–41], attaching the pen to the hand through special devices [42–45], orthoses, using the wrist more than the fingers and optimising the sitting position, general relaxation techniques [46, 47] and general avoidance of stress and anxiety. Writing in private rather than in public may also avoid aggravating stress. Switching the writing hand can be learned within 6–9 months. However, about half of the patients will also develop writer's cramp in the switched hand. Occupational therapy seems to have an adjuvant effect on BT therapy [48]. Figure 4.5 shows a collection of modified pens to enable the patient to cope with writer's cramp.

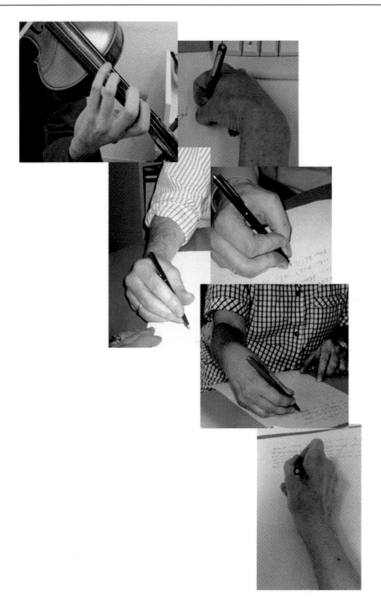

Fig. 4.4 Patients with task-specific dystonia. From: Dressler [74]

Additionally, there are numerous more complicated training programmes, usually referred to as behavioural therapies. This term is used here to describe re-learning processes and not psychotherapeutic techniques. Behavioural therapies include biofeedback techniques [49, 50], often electromyography-based [51–53], habit reversal training [47, 54], constraint-induced motion therapy or sensory motor retuning [55], general training exercises [41, 56–58] and supinator writing practice [40]. Transcranial magnetic brain stimulation has been used experimentally [59].

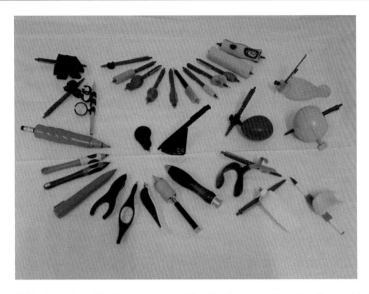

Fig. 4.5 Collection of modified pens to cope with writer's cramp. Photo kindly provided by Mr Arne Knutzen, Kiel, Germany

Musician's dystonia, especially in the forearm and the hand, is treated in a similar manner to writer's cramp. In musician's dystonia the demand for therapy is enormous: most patients use rehabilitation including retraining (87 %), hand therapy (42 %), relaxation techniques (38 %), physiotherapy (30 %), psychotherapy (23 %), acupuncture (21 %) and various body techniques (21 %) [36]. Of the patients, 81.5 % of them report subjective improvement, and around 50 % are estimated to have objective improvement [36].

Simple interventions include ergonomic changes at the instrument [60], changing the grip or the position of the instrument. More complex occupational programmes include behavioural programmes referred to as sensory motor retuning [55, 61–63], sensory training therapy [64–67]), slow-down exercises [68], sensory re-education [69], mixed treatment strategies [70, 71] and immobilisation programmes [72, 73]. Strategies for the prevention of musician's dystonia have been discussed. They include more relaxed positions and stress avoidance. Interestingly, playing jazz music rather than classical music bears a substantially lower risk of dystonia.

Non-focal Dystonia

Figure 4.6 shows a patient with generalised dystonia after central nervous system trauma. Primary treatment for non-focal dystonia depends on the severity and localisation of dystonia [3]. Recently, it was demonstrated that total BT doses can be substantially higher than previously thought [74]. BT therapy can therefore be an alternative in patients previously considered candidates for DBS. It should be directed towards those symptoms generating the highest burden of disease for the

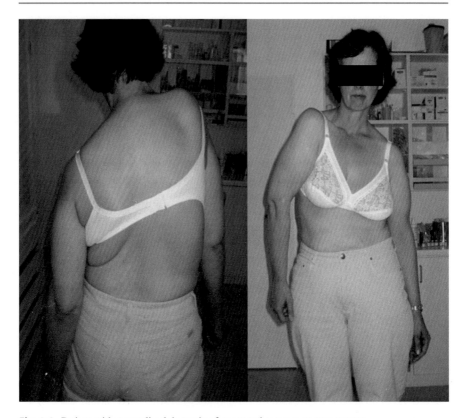

Fig. 4.6   Patient with generalised dystonia after central nervous system trauma

patients. In more severely affected patients and in patients with severe non-focal dystonia DBS becomes the treatment of choice.

Rehabilitation of non-focal dystonia is focussed on those functions most relevant to the patient. It may include use of the hands, walking, swallowing and positioning. Devices to support these functions are frequently used.

References

1. Albanese A, Bhatia K, Bressman SB, Delong MR, Fahn S, Fung VS, Hallett M, Jankovic J, Jinnah HA, Klein C, Lang AE, Mink JW, Teller JK. Phenomenology and classification of dystonia: a consensus update. Mov Disord. 2013;28:863–73.
2. Dressler D, Altenmueller E, Bhidayasiri R, Boholega S, Chana P, Chung TM, Frucht S, Garcia-Ruiz PJ, Kaelin A, Kaji R, Kanovsky P, Laskawi R, Micheli F, Orlova O, Relja M, Rosales R, Slawek J, Timerbaeva S, Warner TT, Adib Saberi F. Strategies for treatment of dystonia. J Neural Transm. 2015;123:251–8.
3. Dressler D, Adib Saberi F, Kollewe K, Schrader C. Safety aspects of incobotulinumtoxinA high dose therapy. J Neural Transm. 2014;122:327–33.

4. Bertrand CM. Selective peripheral denervation for spasmodic torticollis: surgical technique, results, and observation in 260 cases. Surg Neurol. 1993;40:96–103.
5. Dressler D, Berweck S, Chatzikalfas A, Ebke M, Frank B, Hesse S, Huber M, Krauss JK, Mücke K-H, Nolte A, Oelmann H-D, Schönle PW, Schmutzler M, Pickenbrock H, Van der Ven C, Veelken N, Vogel M, Vogt T, Adib Saberi F. Intrathecal baclofen therapy in Germany: proceedings of the IAB-interdisciplinary working group for movement disorders consensus meeting. J Neural Transm. 2015;122:1573–9.
6. Adib Saberi F, Dressler D. Interdisziplinärer Arbeitskreis Bewegungsstörungen (IAB): a new approach for promoting interdisciplinary therapy of movement disorders. J Neural Transm. 2013;120:705–10.
7. Delnooz CC, Horstink MW, Tijssen MA, van de Warrenburg BP. Paramedical treatment in primary dystonia: a systematic review. Mov Disord. 2009;24:2187–98.
8. Bleton JP. Cervical dystonia: a physiotherapy handbook. Paris: Frison Roche; 2014.
9. Counsell C, Sinclair H, Fowlie J, Tyrrell E, Derry N, Meager P, Norrie J, Grosset D. A randomized trial of specialized versus standard neck physiotherapy in cervical dystonia. Parkinsonism Relat Disord. 2016;23:72–9.
10. Ramdharry G. Case report: physiotherapy cuts the dose of botulinum toxin. Physiother Res Int. 2006;11:117–1122.
11. Tassorelli C, Mancini F, Balloni L, Pacchetti C, Sandrini G, Nappi G, Martignoni E. Botulinum toxin and neuromotor rehabilitation: an integrated approach to idiopathic cervical dystonia. Mov Disord. 2006;21:2240–3.
12. Brudny J, Grynbaum BB, Korein J. Spasmodic torticollis: treatment by feedback display of the EMG. Arch Phys Med Rehabil. 1974;55:403–8.
13. Cleeland CS. Behavioral technics in the modification of spasmodic torticollis. Neurology. 1973;1973(23):1241–7.
14. Duddy J. Lack of influence of EMG feedback in relaxation training for spasmodic torticollis. Clin Rehabil. 1995;9:297–303.
15. Harrison DW, Garrett JC, Henderson D, Adams HE. Visual and auditory feedback for head tilt and torsion in a spasmodic torticollis patient. Behav Res Ther. 1985;23:87–8.
16. Jahanshahi M, Sartory G, Marsden CD. EMG biofeedback treatment of torticollis: a controlled outcome study. Biofeedback Self Regul. 1991;16:413–48.
17. Korein J, Brudny J. Integrated EMG feedback in the management of spasmodic torticollis and focal dystonia: a prospective study of 80 patients. Res Publ Assoc Res Nerv Ment Dis. 1976;55:385–426.
18. Leplow B. Heterogeneity of biofeedback training effects in spasmodic torticollis: a single-case approach. Behav Res Ther. 1990;28:359–65.
19. Spencer J, Goetsch VL, Brugnoli RJ, Herman S. Behavior therapy for spasmodic torticollis: a case study suggesting a causal role for anxiety. J Behav Ther Exp Psychiatry. 1991;22:305–11.
20. Andrews HB, Gill HS. Torticollis and serendipity. Arch Phys Med Rehabil. 1982;63:238–9.
21. Faircloth S, Reid S. A cognitive-behavioural approach to the management of idiopathic cervical dystonia. J Behav Ther Exp Psychiatry. 2006;37:239–46.
22. Turner SM, Hersen M, Alford H. Effects of massed practice and meprobamate on spasmodic torticollis: an experimental analysis. Behav Res Ther. 1974;12:259–60.
23. Karnath HO, Konczak J, Dichgans J. Effect of prolonged neck muscle vibration on lateral head tilt in severe spasmodic torticollis. J Neurol Neurosurg Psychiatry. 2000;69:658–60.
24. Leis AA, Dimitrijevic MR, Delapasse JS, Sharkey PC. Modification of cervical dystonia by selective sensory stimulation. J Neurol Sci. 1992;110:79–89.
25. Rosengren SM, Colebatch JG. Cervical dystonia responsive to acoustic and galvanic vestibular stimulation. Mov Disord. 2006;21:1495–9.
26. Cavanaugh JA, Platt JV. Retrocollis: management with orthoplast adapted orthosis. Arch Phys Med Rehabil. 1976;57:300–2.
27. Karapantzou C, Dressler D, Rohrbach S, Laskawi R (2014) Frontalis suspension surgery to treat patients with essential blepharospasm and apraxia of eyelid opening: technique and results. J Plastic Reconstr Aesthet Surg 10:44.

28. Bertolotti G. Biofeedback (BFB) in blepharospasm: two case reports. Appl Psychophysiol Biofeedback. 2005;30:179–80.
29. Brantley PJ, Carnrike Jr CL, Faulstich ME, Barkemeyer CA. Blepharospasm: a case study comparison of trihexyphenidyl (Artane) versus EMG biofeedback. Biofeedback Self Regul. 1985;10:173–80.
30. Peck DF. The use of EMG feedback in the treatment of a severe case of blepharospasm. Biofeedback Self Regul. 1977;2:273–7.
31. Rowan GE, Sedlacek K. Biofeedback in the treatment of blepharospasm: a case study. Am J Psychiatry. 1981;138:1487–9.
32. Roxanas MR, Thomas MR, Rapp MS. Biofeedback treatment of blepharospasm with spasmodic torticollis. Can Med Assoc J. 1978;119:48–9.
33. Stephenson NL. Successful treatment of blepharospasm with relaxation training and biofeedback. Biofeedback Self Regul. 1976;1:331.
34. Blitzer A, Brin MF, Fahn S, Lovelace RE. Clinical and laboratory characteristics of focal laryngeal dystonia: study of 110 cases. Laryngoscope. 1988;98:636–40.
35. Murry T, Woodson GE. Combined-modality treatment of adductor spasmodic dysphonia with botulinum toxin and voice therapy. J Voice. 1995;9:460–5.
36. van Vugt FT, Boullet L, Jabusch HC, Altenmüller E. Musician's dystonia in pianists: long-term evaluation of retraining and other therapies. Parkinsonism Relat Disord. 2014;20:8–12.
37. Bleton JP. Physiotherapy of focal dystonia: a physiotherapist's personal experience. Eur J Neurol. 2010;17 Suppl 1:107–12.
38. Baur B, Schenk T, Fürholzer W, Scheuerecker J, Marquardt C, Kerkhoff G, Hermsdörfer J. Modified pen grip in the treatment of writer's cramp. Hum Mov Sci. 2006;25:464–73.
39. Baur B, Fürholzer W, Jasper I, Marquardt C, Hermsdörfer J. Effects of modified pen grip and handwriting training on writer's cramp. Arch Phys Med Rehabil. 2009;90:867–75.
40. Gupta SK. Behavioural management of writer's cramp: a review of the research evidence. Int J Psychol Psychiatry. 2014;2:126–39.
41. Schenk T, Bauer B, Steidle B, Marquardt C. Does training improve writer's cramp? An evaluation of a behavioral treatment approach using kinematic analysis. J Hand Ther. 2004;17:349–63.
42. Espay AJ, Hung SW, Sanger TD, Moro E, Fox SH, Lang AE. A writing device improves writing in primary writing tremor. Neurology. 2005;64:1648–50.
43. Koller WC, Vetere-Overfield B. Usefulness of a writing aid in writer's cramp. Neurology. 1989;39:149–50.
44. Ranawaya R, Lang A. Usefulness of a writing device in writer's cramp. Neurology. 1991; 41:1136–8.
45. Taş N, Karataş GK, Sepici V. Hand orthosis as a writing aid in writer's cramp. Mov Disord. 2001;16:1185–9.
46. Jacobson E. Progressive relaxation. Chicago: University of Chicago Press; 1938.
47. Wieck A, Harrington R, Marks I, Marsden CD. Writer's cramp: a controlled trial of habit reversal treatment. Br J Psychiatry. 1988;153:111–15.
48. Berg D, Naumann M, Elferich B, Reiners K. Botulinum toxin and occupational therapy in the treatment of writer's cramp. Neurorehabilitation. 1999;12:169–76.
49. Baur B, Fürholzer W, Marquardt C, Hermsdörfer J. Auditory grip force feedback in the treatment of Writer's Cramp. J Hand Ther. 2009;22:163–70.
50. O'Neill MA, Gwinn KA, Adler CH. Biofeedback for writer's cramp. Am J Occup Ther. 1997;51:605–7.
51. Bindman E, Tibbetts RW. Writer's Cramp—a rational approach to treatment? Br J Psychiatry. 1977;131:143–8.
52. Cottraux JA, Juenet C, Collet L. The treatment of writer's cramp with multimodal behaviour therapy and biofeedback: a study of 15 cases. Br J Psychiatry. 1983;142:180–3.
53. Deepak KK, Behari M. Specific muscle EMG biofeedback for hand dystonia. Appl Psychophysiol Biofeedback. 1999;24:267–80.

54. Greenberg D. Writer's cramp—a habit for reversal? J Behav Ther Exp Psychiatry. 1983;14:233–9.
55. Candia V, Rosset-Llobet J, Elbert T, Pascual-Leone A. Changing the brain through therapy for musicians' hand dystonia. Ann N Y Acad Sci. 2005;1060:335–42.
56. Mai N, Marquardt C. Schreibtraining in der neurologischen Rehabilitation. In: EKN-Materialien für die Rehabilitation. Borgmann: Dortmund; 1999.
57. Marquardt C, Mai N. Treatment of writer's cramp: kinematic measures as assessment tools for planning and evaluating handwriting training procedures. In: Fausc C, Keuss P, Vinler G, editors. Advances in handwriting and drawing. Paris: Europia; 1994. p. 445–61.
58. Zeuner KE, Shill HA, Sohn YH, Molloy FM, Thornton BC, Dambrosia JM, Hallett M. Motor training as treatment in focal hand dystonia. Mov Disord. 2005;20:335–41.
59. Kimberley TJ, Borich MR, Schmidt RL, Carey JR, Gillick B. Focal hand dystonia: individualized intervention with repeated application of repetitive transcranial magnetic stimulation. Arch Phys Med Rehabil. 2015;96(4 Suppl):S122–8.
60. Rosset-Llobet J, Fàbregas i Molas S, Rosinés i Cubells D, Narberhaus Donner B, Montero i Homs J. Clinical analysis of musicians' focal hand dystonia. Review of 86 cases. Neurologia. 2005;20:108–15.
61. Berque P, Gray H, Harkness C, McFadyen A. A combination of constraint-induced therapy and motor control retraining in the treatment of focal hand dystonia in musicians. Med Probl Perform Art. 2010;25:149–61.
62. Candia V, Elbert T, Altenmüller E, Rau H, Schäfer T, Taub E. Constraint-induced movement therapy for focal hand dystonia in musicians. Lancet. 1999;353(9146):42.
63. Candia V, Schäfer T, Taub E, Rau H, Altenmüller E, Rockstroh B, Elbert T. Sensory motor retuning: a behavioral treatment for focal hand dystonia of pianists and guitarists. Arch Phys Med Rehabil. 2002;83:1342–8.
64. Byl NN, Nagarajan SS, Merzenich MM, Roberts T, McKenzie A. Correlation of clinical neuromusculoskeletal and central somatosensory performance: variability in controls and patients with severe and mild focal hand dystonia. Neural Plast. 2002;9(3):177–203.
65. Byl NN, Nagajaran S, McKenzie AL. Effect of sensory discrimination training on structure and function in patients with focal hand dystonia: a case series. Arch Phys Med Rehabil. 2003;84(10):1505–14.
66. Byl NN, Archer ES, McKenzie A. Focal hand dystonia: effectiveness of a home program of fitness and learning-based sensorimotor and memory training. J Hand Ther. 2009;22:183–97.
67. Zeuner KE, Bara-Jimenez W, Noguchi PS, Goldstein SR, Dambrosia JM, Hallett M. Sensory training for patients with focal hand dystonia. Ann Neurol. 2002;51:593–8.
68. Sakai N. Slow-down exercise for the treatment of focal hand dystonia in pianists. Med Probl Perf Artists. 2006;21:25–8.
69. Chaná-Cuevas P, Kunstmann-Rioseco C, Rodríguez-Riquelme T. Guitarist's cramp: management with sensory re-education. Rev Neurol. 2003;37:637–40.
70. Jabusch HC, Zschucke D, Schmidt A, Schuele S, Altenmüller E. Focal dystonia in musicians: treatment strategies and long-term outcome in 144 patients. Mov Disord. 2005;20:1623–6.
71. Schuele SU, Lederman RJ. Long-term outcome of focal dystonia in instrumental musicians. Adv Neurol. 2004;94:261–6.
72. Pesenti A, Barbieri S, Priori A. Limb immobilization for occupational dystonia: a possible alternative treatment for selected patients. Adv Neurol. 2004;94:247–54.
73. Priori A, Pesenti A, Cappellari A, Scarlato G, Barbieri S. Limb immobilization for the treatment of focal occupational dystonia. Neurology. 2001;57:405–9.
74. Dressler D. Botulinumtoxin-Therapie: ein Ratgeber für Patienten. Hamburg: IAB; 2015.

Rehabilitation of Ataxia

5

Marise Bueno Zonta, Giovana Diaferia, José Luiz Pedroso, and Hélio A.G. Teive

Introduction

Cerebellar ataxias represent an extensive group of heterogeneous diseases, characterized by gait impairment and loss of balance, used related to cerebellar involvement. There are several forms of cerebellar ataxias, including acute causes (for instance, cerebellar stroke) or neurodegenerative disorders (such as hereditary ataxias). There is no effective treatment for the hereditary ataxias, and management remains supportive and symptomatic. For acute cerebellar syndrome, rehabilitation is mandatory. Rehabilitation process may lead to improvement in cerebellar symptoms and daily life functions, and must be included as a crucial treatment option for the cerebellar ataxias.

Motor Rehabilitation

Rehabilitation is essential for all patients with ataxia. Any approach that includes physical therapy can help to improve quality of life. Physical therapy should start early at the diagnosis of ataxia, even in people with mild symptoms, such as sporadic imbalance. Therapy on the ground should consist of balance training and therapists may suggest other practices that are complementary to the treatment program. When people present with the early signs and symptoms of ataxia, they are likely to engage in unsupervised activities in an attempt to minimize their symptoms. Guidance of a skilled professional is key at the beginning of any program to

M.B. Zonta, P.T., Ph.D. • H.A.G. Teive, M.D., Ph.D.
Universidade Federal do Paraná, Curitiba, PR, Brazil

G. Diaferia, S.L.P., M.Sc. • J.L. Pedroso, M.D., Ph.D. (✉)
Department of Neurology, Universidade Federal de São Paulo, São Paulo, Brazil
e-mail: gidiaferia@hotmail.com; zeluizpedroso@yahoo.com.br

© Springer International Publishing Switzerland 2017
H.F. Chien, O.G.P. Barsottini (eds.), *Movement Disorders Rehabilitation*,
DOI 10.1007/978-3-319-46062-8_5

incorporate activities that are suitable for these patients. In general, patients with ataxia should be encouraged to exercise as part of health promotion, and as long as risk factors and safety considerations have been assessed. Exercise should be tailored individually and may involve exploring several different options for building motivation, but patients with ataxia should be fully aware of the importance of motor coordination and balance training.

Physical therapy should not be discontinued in advanced stages of disease in dependent, bedridden people because passive/assisted mobilization and correct positioning are essential at these stages to maintain the same level of residual activity, prevent pain and bedsores, and improve well-being. Over the course of the disease, management targets should be adjusted based on the patient's health status and needs taking into account individual characteristics, including age, interests, and financial resources, among others.

Rehabilitation of patients with ataxia involves a thorough assessment to establish the patient's current level of functioning and to set up treatment goals and strategies. Regular reassessments are also necessary to assess the effectiveness of the current management and to identify any changes to the treatment plan that may be required [1].

Patients with ataxia have specific needs depending on their symptoms. Individually tailored physical therapy strategies should be planned and incorporate specific objectives and goals toward the highest possible level of functioning, with continuous adjustments over time to minimize loss of function. Besides motor coordination and balance training, other goals can be set, including increased transfer and locomotion independence; muscle strengthening; increased physical resilience; "safe fall" strategy; learning to use mobility aids (e.g., a walker); learning how to reduce the body's energy expenditure; developing specific breathing patterns; monitoring posture while sitting and standing; preventing and minimizing deformities and pain in people confined to a bed and/or wheelchair; and learning muscle relaxation exercises, among others [2]. Patient assessment can provide objective information to guide the use of these therapy modalities or a combination of different modalities.

In their review, Cassidy et al. [3] make recommendations on physical therapy interventions, including dynamic task practices that challenge stability and explore stability limits; combined strength and flexibility training; a compensatory approach including orthotics and devices; teaching practical, everyday strategies for those with severe upper extremity tremor; and careful documentation of patient outcomes.

A physical therapy plan should be prepared from the interpretation of the assessment results and can vary depending on the type and characteristics of ataxia [1]. Recovery of motor function depends on the cause and the site of the cerebellar injury [4]. Although approaches that improve proprioception and incorporate visual aids are used more commonly in people with sensory ataxia, stabilization training is more important to reduce truncal and extremity ataxia in people with cerebellar ataxia. People with vestibular ataxia should be given habituation exercises to reduce vertigo, and vestibulo-ocular and vestibulospinal reflexes should be stimulated to improve balance. In some challenging cases, such as mixed ataxia, a number of physical therapy interventions are required. When preparing a treatment plan, it should be kept in mind that the proprioceptive, vestibular, and visual systems and the cerebellum are closely related, and that balance and coordination result from this relationship [1]. These authors argue that the methods applied for the rehabilitation of ataxia cannot be classified as approaches directed merely toward proprioception or balance, as all of these interact with each other.

Physical therapy techniques may vary depending on the approach used. An individual treatment may consist of modalities on the ground (with or without equipment), and/or in the water (hydrotherapy), and/or on a horse (equine therapy), and/or virtual reality training. In a single exercise practice or therapy session they can work stability, balance, strength, elongation, and motor coordination at the same time as all these skills are interconnected.

Regarding motor recovery, two major issues have deserved attention in the rehabilitation of degenerative cerebellar diseases [5]. The first issue is whether motor sequence learning or relearning of everyday tasks occurs, as the cerebellum plays a crucial role in motor learning. The second one is whether gains in motor function can be maintained over time given the progressive nature of these conditions. Ilg et al. [4] contend that motor rehabilitation in people with cerebellar damage is challenging because the cerebellum plays an important role in motor learning and they may have difficulty recovering function with physical therapy owing to damage to structures critically involved in the relearning of motor skills.

In another review, Ilg et al. [4] looked at studies that assessed physical therapy interventions for patients with cerebellar ataxia. These interventions included progressive stimulation on gait and balance for improved postural stability and less dependence in daily life activities. The authors note that most studies comprised heterogeneous, small samples, making it difficult to compare the methods of intervention. They also cite the clinical studies by Ilg et al. [6] and Miyail et al. [5], both large cohorts that systematically showed the benefits of motor rehabilitation in patients with cerebellar degenerative diseases. Ilg et al. [7] found significant benefits of intensive coordination and balance training that persisted over 12 months, despite a gradual decline in motor performance due to progressive neurodegenerative symptoms.

The finding that patients with ataxia can improve movement performance [6] corroborated that seen in physical therapy practice. Therapists' current challenge is to find new ways to encourage patients to keep up with continuous training to preserve their gains. Continuous coordination and balance training should be the standard of care; however, raising patient awareness and adjusting their daily routine are required. An exercise program should take into account patient age, clinical features, and prognosis. There are countless exercises available and a good therapist should find new creative ways to keep patients interested and engaged.

The physical therapy approaches listed in a review study by Armutlu [1] are designed for proprioception improvement, balance and stabilization training, and vertigo and dizziness reduction. The author reviewed several studies on approaches to improving proprioception that included techniques to increase proprioception input through mechanical stimulation of articular surfaces, muscles, and tendons, decreasing postural instability by improving body awareness. The techniques include proprioceptive neuromuscular facilitation (PNF), mat activities, resistive exercises, use of Johnstone pressure splints, gait exercises on different surfaces (hard, soft, and inclined surfaces) with eyes open and closed, and vibration techniques. They also included body awareness and balance activities. The authors of the studies reviewed cited exercise disciplines such as Tai Chi and yoga. Proximal stabilization and activities in different positions with movement progress from one position to another were emphasized. These authors concur that the best indicator of dynamic stabilization and balance is gait.

Frenkel exercises were also developed for the stimulation of proprioception. Simon Frenkel (1860–1931) was a pioneer of neurorehabilitation and developed an exercise program with various positions for improving motor coordination, balance, and therefore ataxia. These exercises can be used in combination with PNF techniques [8] and both are effective in mild cases of ataxia.

A variety of physical therapy techniques involves balance and proprioception stimulation. The main principles of therapy are:

1. Keep the best posture for as long as the patient can. For example, people who are able to walk or stand should maintain it for long enough. They should also be encouraged to maintain a "standing position" as home practice (e.g., standing while watching TV for a period every day, even if they need support). The focus is to preserve their level of functioning: if a person is able to walk, she/he should do it as much as possible. The order of exercises does not matter; it is important to exercise as many positions as possible by using different mechanisms and muscles, giving emphasis to the best posture.
2. Promote stability by using different positions and while progressing from one position to another. Train both static postural stability and dynamic postural stability for every position. Mechanical stimulation of joint surfaces, muscles, and tendons increases sensory and proprioceptive information on these body areas and helps reduce instability.
3. In addition to balance and coordination exercises, muscle strength and stretching exercises should be performed in every position. Some people may require stretching exercises at the beginning of the therapy session, whereas others may gradually change positions and progressively perform stretching exercises.
4. Balance training should be functional, i.e., people should practice functions in the performance of daily tasks that require balance and proper posture. Improving posture control will promote a maximum level of functional capacity; training may help to reduce postural sway during movement.
5. As patients have to maintain an unbalanced position to train balance reactions, these exercises should be performed safely and progress depending on their symptoms. The degree of difficulty of an exercise should gradually be increased using obstacles or provoking balance reactions to challenge them in a safe exercise routine.
6. Strength training should use body weight exercises. Building muscle strength is crucial, but care should be taken not to fatigue the muscles. It is important to

strengthen proximal shoulder and hip muscles to maintain the function of the upper and lower extremities.

7. Exercises should be practiced consciously at first, and in later stages should be followed by automatic exercise activities. Exercises should progress from simple to complex within people's functional level bearing in mind symptom progression. Some exercises should be practiced first with the eyes open and later with the eyes closed.

8. A home practice program should incorporate other physical activities such as sport activities to train components of basic skills in patients with ataxia. They should be provided with support materials with pictures/drawings to guide their home exercise routine [9].

Use of Virtual Reality Applications

Intensive balance and motor coordination training can make people weary and be a complex practice for children with ataxia especially those lacking motivation. A major advantage of virtual reality is to motivate patients. The literature also reports additional benefits including improved balance and posture, locomotion and gait, and upper and lower extremity function [10, 11].

Many researchers point out the potential of virtual reality games as an effective approach to improve motor skills and as a tool for assessing treatment effectiveness. They have investigated a broad variety of therapeutic applications, especially for motor and locomotor function rehabilitation in patients with neurological conditions, and in patients with cognitive impairment. Ilg et al. [10] assessed the effectiveness of using three X-Box® videogame sets in children with ataxia. The children underwent an 8-week training program (2 weeks at the study site and 6 weeks in their homes) specifically designed to improve motor coordination and balance. The authors found that videogames reduced symptoms of ataxia, improved the children's ability to maintain good balance, and made the step-to-step transition while walking safer and more effective.

Vestibular Rehabilitation Exercises

People with secondary, nongenetic, and hereditary degenerative ataxia have vestibular complaints in daily clinical practice that require treatment. Different vestibular rehabilitation protocols are available and each has distinctive characteristics. The Cawthorne–Cooksey exercise protocol (1946) was designed to treat vestibular ataxia. This exercise program is aimed at reducing vestibular disturbances, including vertigo, vision changes during head motions, and balance and motor problems. It consists of a series of head movements, body movements, and head–eye coordination and balance exercises performed in various positions where patients are instructed to perform the exercises slowly at first, and then increasing speed. These exercises are intended to improve the patient's well-being while performing daily activities. In his review [1],

Armutlu cites some studies that show the use of many components of this exercise program by physical therapists and occupational therapists.

Many protocols [12] are available to treat people with vestibular ataxia, in particular those using virtual reality applications. Virtual reality-based vestibular rehabilitation consists of interactive graphics creating a virtual reality experience [13]. The benefits of this treatment are reported in the literature and include balance and posture alignment, improved mobility and upper and lower extremity function, and increased motivation to exercise.

Vestibular rehabilitation exercises, either conventional or virtual reality-based protocols, have the same goal of seeking to restore body balance, stimulating and accelerating the natural mechanisms of vestibular compensation, and thus enhancing neuroplasticity in people with peripheral and/or central vestibular disorders. The sole difference is the equipment used to achieve vestibular compensation.

Adding Extra Weight to Exercises

Weighted anklets attached to lower extremities, vests to be worn on the trunk, belts around the waist, cuffs, and adapted insoles to be placed in shoes can be used to add extra weight to exercises. Better movement control is expected. A study by Dias et al. [14] showed the effectiveness of adding extra weight to exercise to improve static postural balance and dynamic postural balance, gait coordination, and functional independence. This finding is corroborated by that reported by providers and patients training with extra weights and suggests that this practice should be considered on an individual basis.

A few studies have investigated the effect of adding extra weight to exercise in patients with ataxia. These investigations mostly involved small samples of low quality and thus did not provide any strong evidence [15, 16]. In the review by Cassidy et al. 3], the authors question adding extra weight when performing lower extremity exercises. However, they recommend extra weight to control ataxia in the wrist and hand, and build wrist strength to reduce tremors [17].

Adding extra weight can increase tremors and cause discomfort in patients with ataxia. The need and indication for adding extra weight should be assessed on an individual basis and require skilled supervision.

Sports Activities

In their review studies, Armutlu [1], Cassidy et al. [3], and Synofzik and Ilg [18] underline the importance of sports activities for balance and coordination training. In clinical practice, patients with ataxia should be encouraged to be active, taking their preferences into consideration. While a daily 1-h exercise routine is realistic in research settings because a timeframe is set for this activity, better adherence is likely with a weekly program including different activities in clinical settings. Such a training program may include sports/recreational activities based on people's abilities and interests.

For many people with disabilities, adaptive sports are a way of reestablishing contact with the outside world, and may prove motivating to patients with ataxia. A number of sports activities (hiking, basketball, tennis, ping-pong, volleyball, bowling, swimming, darts, and golf, among others) can be adapted for patients with ataxia. Other activities including Tai Chi, yoga, Qigong, dancing, and Pilates training offer challenging coordination and balance exercises and may motivate people with playful and pleasurable movements. People at the early stage of the disease who are able to go "jogging" or engage in their favorite sports without difficulty should be encouraged to keep practicing for as long as possible.

Prospects for Rehabilitation of Ataxia

Currently, rehabilitation of ataxia basically involves physical therapy, occupational therapy, and speech therapy [4]. Physical therapy not only plays a role in recovering motor function, but also in helping to alleviate respiratory, urinary, ocular, and orthopedic dysfunction that may accompany ataxia. Further investigations with controlled studies and documentation of results are needed.

Recovery of motor function was the subject of a review study by Synofzik and Ilg [18]. Encouraging results were reported that demonstrated that high-intensity motor coordination training offers a significant benefit in patients with degenerative ataxia, with gains in stability and motor coordination. The authors reviewed studies involving both high-intensity therapy training (coordination and balance exercises) and controlled videogame training (exergame training) and found a benefit corresponding to the recovery of one or more years of the natural progression of the disease. Moreover, they suggest that even people in the advanced stages of the disease can benefit from this type of training. Note that in both types of training the effects seem related to the frequency of exercises and maintenance of an ongoing exercise program.

This review study showed that improvements do not result from nonspecific changes, but rather they reflect the recovery of dysfunctions that may accompany ataxia. Even children with severe ataxia can be motivated to engage in a demanding exercise program, as they recover their own movements and experience feelings of success.

In light of the above, the authors introduced a new concept for ataxia training in clinical practice drawing from the notion that rehabilitation in degenerative ataxia should optimally resort to a large array of different training strategies that can be individually tailored according to each individual's ataxia type, disease stage, and personal training preferences.

As for clinical practice recommendations, they suggest different treatment approaches according to the degree of patient involvement [18]. Patients at the very early stages of ataxia should practice demanding sporting exercises that provide great challenges to the coordination system. Real-world sports may be complemented by demanding Xbox Kinect games. These games can be played on an elastic mattress to increase the challenge. As people become more committed to the training program, the role of the physical therapist becomes increasingly important for specific balance training and safety techniques, and games (Kinect games) should be progressively adjusted in addition to any treatment [18].

In conclusion, physical therapy remains challenging for physicians and their rehabilitation teams. They should bear in mind that published research findings are based on means and medians and that it is important to note individual variations among patients. Although the disease undoubtedly has an enormous impact on patient outcomes, they are also dependent on people's will to live, adherence to treatment, the resources available, determination, willingness, and other nonreproducible individual characteristics.

Speech and Voice Therapy in Ataxia

Early symptoms of disease include muscle problems, walking and balance difficulties, involuntary eye movements, and double vision. Different areas and/or functions of the central and/or peripheral nervous system are marked by progressive degeneration, including pathways involved with the motor control of speech and swallowing. As disease progresses, communication skills and deglutition become impaired, requiring the use of alternative resources. Speech therapy interventions are aimed at treating changes in deglutition, as swallowing difficulty can cause aspiration pneumonia in most cases [19].

Interventions targeting mechanical and functional components of deglutition and speech articulation are most effective when these impairments are detected and understood. Studies on changes in speech/voice and deglutition in Machado–Joseph disease (MJD) are scarce, but Wolf et al. [20] investigated changes in speech and voice in ten patients and found imprecise articulation with a slow rate of speech, a hoarse–breathy voice quality, and decreased volume. The authors emphasize that complaints involving communication may not be consistent with objective findings in the clinical evaluation, and thus speech therapists must pay special attention to patients' expectations and communication skills. Difficulty in articulation due to impairment of the neuromuscular control of speech is conventionally called dysarthria. The word derives from the Greek words *dys + arthroun*, meaning the inability to utter distinctly [21]. However, owing to an association with phonation impairment, dysarthrophonia is a more appropriate term.

Dysarthrophonia affects all aspects of speech, including resonance, articulation, phonation, and respiration at different levels of severity and produces different signs. It may be characterized by changes in speech production, emission, articulation, voice, and prosody resulting from cerebellar injury. Gestures are slow, less intense, and imprecise. MJD is characterized by different motor manifestations producing different, poorly described speech and voice patterns.

Dysphagia, or difficulty swallowing, is present in neurodegenerative diseases and is responsible for clinical complications including aspiration pneumonia, which is the most common cause of death in these patients. Dysphagia affects quality of life as it can cause nutritional disturbances, dehydration, lung conditions, and patients may even suffer from a loss of pleasure from eating and social interactions.

Jardim et al. [22] evaluated 62 patients with MJD presenting with dysarthria, muscle fasciculation, pyramidal syndrome, and ophthalmoplegia. They found that the earlier the age of onset, the more severe the progression of MJD, and vice versa [23, 24].

Ataxia patients may have a normal or a hoarse, harsh voice with a strained, strangled quality [25]. Vocal tremor is uncommon in ataxia, but may occur owing to changes in laryngeal and respiratory muscles, and is characteristically irregular and slow [26]. In a study on patients with MJD, Wolf [19] found the presence of a hoarse, breathy, strained vocal quality, hypernasality, and little intraoral air pressure in consonant production. Although the main feature of MJD is ataxia, changes in the pyramidal, extrapyramidal, and peripheral nervous system may determine various voice qualities. When extrapyramidal symptoms are predominant, voice characteristics may be close to those of Parkinson's disease and include reduced volume, monopitch, hoarseness, and a breathy voice quality. Monopitch is a typical feature and is more frequent than high–low pitch variation [27]. Pitch fluctuation in ataxic dysarthria is produced by impaired cerebellar control of the proprioceptive circuit mediated by extracerebellar structures in both laryngeal and respiratory muscles [28]. According to the literature, resonance changes in ataxic dysarthria are uncommon and hyponasality may occur because of impaired temporal control of the soft palate contraction [29]. However, according to Theodoro et al. [30], the rate of hypernasality is high in dysarthria (95 %). The study by Wolf [19] showed that dysarthria in patients with MJD is closer to mixed than to ataxic dysarthria.

Theodoro et al. [30] evaluated 20 subjects with ataxic dysarthria using perceptual and acoustic analysis methods and reported a high rate of hypernasality (95 %). Another study by Kent et al. [31] evaluated 14 subjects with ataxic dysarthria to determine which features of the disorder were most consistent, which speaking tasks were most sensitive to the disorder, and whether the different speech production subsystems were uniformly affected. Perceptual and acoustic data were obtained for several speaking tasks, including sustained vowel phonation, syllable repetition, sentence recitation, and conversation. The most frequent abnormality for both male and female subjects was the variability of the fundamental frequency, followed by shimmer and jitter (short-term frequency and amplitude perturbation). Jitter was more pronounced among females. The syllable alternating motion rate (AMR) was typically slow and irregular. The energy maxima and minima were highly variable across repeated syllables, which reflects poorly coordinated respiratory function and inadequate articulatory and voicing control. Syllable rates tended to be slower for sentence recitation and conversation than for AMR. Conversational samples varied considerably in intelligibility and number of words/morphemes in a breath group among subjects. Qualitative analyses of unintelligible episodes in conversation showed that these samples generally had a well-defined syllable pattern. Schalling et al. [32] evaluated 21 subjects who had spinocerebellar ataxia with mild to moderate dysarthria and 21 controls. Those with ataxic dysarthria demonstrated strained phonation, imprecise consonants, vocal instability, monotony, and a reduced speech rate of syllables per second in repeated syllables. The acoustic analysis showed reduced a reading rate of syllables per second, repetition of syllables, long syllables, and variation in breaks. The authors recommend both acoustic and perceptual analyses for evaluating ataxic individuals.

The study by Wolf [19] reported changes in five prosodic items and rhythm, reduced stress, prolonged intervals, and inadequate breaks. Hence, it is important to assess sound duration. Casper et al. [33] studied subjects with cerebellar ataxia and found significant changes in prosodic items compared with the control group, in addition to changes in sound duration. Spencer and Slocomb [34] reported that patients with cerebellar damage present with abnormal speech articulation and prosody. Regarding speech articulation, patients with MJD show imprecise articulation, prolongation, repetition, interruptions between sounds, distortion of vowels, and an irregular and slow rate of repetition of syllables [19]. Portnoy and Aronson [35] investigated three groups of 30 subjects each: a normal group; a group with ataxic dysarthria; and a group with spastic dysarthria. Using a computer, they measured by a diadochokinetic syllable rate for /p/, /t/, and /k/. The normal group showed syllable rates per second of 6.4 for /p/, 6.1 for /t/, and 5.7 for /k/. Subjects with ataxic dysarthria showed rates of 3.8, 3.9, and 3.4, and those with spastic dysarthria showed rates of 4.6, 4.2, and 3.5 respectively. The slow rate of repetition in the ataxic subjects and the significantly more variable rhythm of repetition in the spastic subjects were unexpected findings and are in contrast to results from perceptual analysis. The study demonstrates that slowness of syllable repetition is not restricted to spastic dysarthria and that dysrhythmia of syllable repetition is not restricted to ataxic dysarthria. They point to the importance of operationalizing measurements. Padovani et al. [36] compared normal subjects with individuals with neurological disorders and reported statistically significant differences in the production of all syllables. Diadochokinesia was increasingly different in the two groups as sound production moved from the outermost articulatory point, i.e., the bilabial phoneme, to the innermost point, i.e., the larynx. The articulatory and laryngeal diadochokinesia test proved to be sensitive to differentiating the normal group from the subjects with dysarthria. It underscores the importance of incorporating this test into speech–language evaluation protocols to look for neuromotor integrity abnormalities and help differential diagnosis and monitoring of progressive diseases, especially in patients with laryngeal dystonia, amyotrophic lateral sclerosis, bulbar symptoms, and ataxia.

Several studies have investigated diadochokinesia, as it involves consecutive articulatory movements, and the ability to perform rapid repetitions of simple speech segments is an indicator of sound speed of articulatory movements and points of articulation. It is thus a neurological skill test that shows the adequacy of neuromotor maturation and integration [37].

Dysphagia is common in individuals with MJD; however, few studies have investigated its occurrence. An epidemiological, clinical, and pathological study reported that dysphagia occurs from year 8 of disease onset in 70 % of patients and that from year 15 it becomes moderate or severe and may cause death from tracheobronchial aspiration, bronchopneumonia, or malnutrition because of the difficulty swallowing [38]. Younger age is associated with earlier and more severe symptoms of voice, speech, and swallowing problems [20]. Patients with degenerative ataxia have greater difficulty swallowing liquids than solid foods, and penetration is significantly higher for liquids than solid foods. Greater difficulty swallowing liquids may be due to a delayed swallowing response and liquids may either reach the epiglottis before it closes or inundate the epiglottis before the movement is complete [39].

Studies have suggested that a delayed swallow reflex [40] might result in decreased pharyngeal contraction movements and reduced glottal efficiency, i.e., stasis of food in the valleculae and piriform sinuses, in addition to the risk of penetration and aspiration. In a study of 33 patients with MJD, Wolf [19] found that increased food viscosity and volume was related to greater stasis of food, especially in the valleculae and piriform sinuses. Posterior intraoral escape of food was only significantly higher when examined by increasing liquid viscosity from 3 mL of liquid to 3 mL of honey. Wolf also observed stasis of food in the valleculae with 3 mL of honey and a posterior escape of 5 mL of honey, with values close to 1.0 (not significant). In addition, laryngeal penetration was statistically significant with increased viscosity from honey to pudding, which suggests difficulties with the motor control of the laryngeal musculature with poor airway protection. Abnormal oral motor control in subjects with MJD explains the increased swallowing difficulty of larger bolus volumes and increased bolus viscosity, which increases the stasis of food and episodes of penetration, as the swallowing process depends on a pump mechanism, according to Costa [41].

Despite the scarcity of investigations into swallowing in patients with MJD, the studies available have reported greater difficulty experienced swallowing liquids than solids [39]. Contrasting with findings by Rüb et al. [23] of gradual improvement in swallowing with increased bolus viscosity, Wolf [19] showed worsening of symptoms as the bolus volume and viscosity increased. Abnormal oral motor control of greater bolus volume and viscosity probably causes premature escape of food [41, 42]. Another study by Diaféria et al. [43] reported the main findings of fiber optic endoscopic evaluation of swallowing (FEES) in patients with MJD, including stasis in the piriform sinuses and posterior pharyngeal wall, stasis in the valleculae after ingestion of paste-like food with a thick consistency, residue on the tongue base, and stasis in the posterior pharyngeal wall after ingestion of thickened liquids. They did not find penetration and tracheolaryngeal aspiration before or after swallowing across all consistencies. Patients with MJD show abnormalities of the oral and pharyngeal stages of swallowing owing to oral motor control impairment, making it difficult to swallow high bolus volumes and viscosities in the oral cavity, and thus increasing food stasis. Endoscopy swallow images have been shown to be an effective tool in the diagnosis of oropharyngeal dysphagia in patients with MJD.

Drawing on these findings, it can be assumed that increased bolus viscosity and volume have a less significant effect on oral motor control in patients with MJD. Further studies on speech articulation and swallowing may improve our knowledge on this chronic progressive disease so that patients can maintain communication as far as possible at every stage of their disease, in addition to preserving social interaction and increasing swallowing safety to prevent complications such as aspiration and malnutrition.

Quality of life and longevity of patients with ataxia depends on the appropriate treatment of motor symptoms and continuous multidisciplinary monitoring by a team composed of a physical therapist, a speech therapist, a psychologist, and an occupational therapist. In particular, long-term speech–language therapy may result in language improvement.

References

 1. Armutlu, K. Ataxia: physical therapy and rehabilitation applications for ataxic patients. Buffalo University, 2010. Disponível em: http://www.cirrie.buffalo.edu/encyclopedia/en/article/112/.
 2. Fonteyn EM, Keus SH, Verstappen CC, et al. The effectiveness of allied health care in patients with ataxia: a systematic review. J Neurol. 2014;261(2):251–8.
 3. Cassidy E, Kilbride C, Holland A. Management of the ataxias: towards best clinical practice—physiotherapy supplement. London: Ataxia UK; 2009.
 4. Ilg W, et al. Consensus paper: management of degenerative cerebellar disorders. Cerebellum. 2014;13:248–68. doi:10.1007/s12311-013-0531-6.
 5. Miyail IM, Hattori N, Mihara M, Hatakenaka M, Yagura H, et al. Cerebellar ataxia rehabilitation trial in degenerative cerebellar diseases. Neurorehabil Neural Repair. 2012;26:515–22.
 6. Ilg W, Synofzik M, Brotz D, Burkard S, Giese MA, Schols L. Intensive coordinative training improves motor performance in degenerative cerebellar disease. Neurology. 2009;73:1823–30.
 7. Ilg W, Brötz D, Burkard S, Giese MA, Schöls L, Synofzik M. Long term effects of coordinative training in degenerative cerebellar disease. Mov Disord. 2010;25:2239–46.
 8. Armutlu K, Karabudak R, Nurlu G. Physiotherapy approaches in the treatment of ataxic multiple sclerosis: a pilot study. Neurorehabil Neural Repair. 2001;15:203–11.
 9. Zonta MB, Silva RM, Teive HAG. Fisioterapia nas Ataxias—Manual para o paciente. Disponível em: http://www.hc.ufpr.br/reabilitacao.
10. Ilg WI, Schatton C, Schicks J, Giese M, Schöls L, Synofzik M. Video game–based coordinative training improves ataxia in children with degenerative ataxia. Neurology. 2012;79(20):2056–60.
11. Synofzik M, Schatton C, Giese M, et al. Videogame-based coordinative training can improve advanced, multisystemic early-onset ataxia. J Neurol. 2013;260(10):2656–8.
12. Dannenbaum E, Rappaport JM, Paquet N, Visitim M, Fung J, Watt D. Year review of a novel vestibular rehabilitation program in Montreal and Laval, Quebec. J Otolaryngol. 2004;33(1):5–9.
13. Zeigelboim BS, Souza SD, Mengelberg H, Teive HAG, Santos RS, Liberalesso PBN. Reabilitação vestibular com realidade virtual na ataxia espinocerebelar. Audiol Commun Res. 2013;18(2):143–7.
14. Dias ML, Toti F, Almeida SRM, Oberg TD. Efeito do peso para membros inferiores no equilíbrio estático e dinâmico nos portadores de ataxia. Acta Fisiatr. 2009;16(3):116–20.
15. Clopton N, Schultz D, Boren C, Porter J, Brillhart T. Effects of axial loading on gait for subjects with cerebellar ataxia: preliminary findings. Neurol Rep. 2003;27:15–21.
16. Gibson-Horn C. Balance-based torso-weighting in a patient with ataxia and multiple sclerosis: a case report. J Neurol Phys Ther. 2008;32:139–46.
17. Mcgrunder J, Cors D, Tiernan AM, Tomlin G. Weighted wrist cuffs for tremor reduction during eating in adults with static brain lesions. Am J Occup Ther. 2003;57:507–16.
18. Synofzik M, Ilg W. Motor training in degenerative spinocerebellar disease: ataxia-specific improvements by intensive physiotherapy and exergames. Biomed Res Int. 2014;2014, 583507. doi:10.1155/2014/583507.
19. Wolf, AE. Aspectos clínicos da deglutição, da fonoarticulação e suas correlações genéticas na doença de Machado Joseph/Aline Epiphanio Wolf. Campinas, SP: [s.n.], 2008.
20. Wolf A, Santos D, Canadas N, Medeiros R, Sales T, Quagliato E, Viana M, Crespo A. Alterações fonoaudiológicas na Doença de Machado–Joseph. Santos: Trabalho apresentado como pôster no XII Congresso Brasileiro de Fonoaudiologia; 2005.
21. Darley FL, Aronson AE, Brown JR. Clusters of deviant speech dimensions in the dysarthrias. J Speech Hear Res. 1969;12:462–96.
22. Jardim LB, Pereira ML, Silveira I, Ferro A, Sequeiros J, Giugliarri R. Neurologic findings in Machado-Joseph disease. Arch Neurol. 2001;58(6):899–904.
23. Rüb U, Brunt ER, Del Turco D, de Vos RA, Gierga K, Paulson H, Braak H. Guidelines for the pathoanatomical examination of the lower brain stem in ingestive and swallowing disorders

and its application to a dysphagic spinocerebellar ataxia type 3 patient. Neuropathol Appl Neurobiol. 2003;29(1):1–13.

24. Maruyama H, Nakamura S, Matsuyama Z, Sakai T, Doyu M, Sobue G, Seto M, Tsujihata M, Oh-i T, Nishio T. Molecular features of the CAG repeats and clinical manifestation of Machado-Joseph disease. Hum Mol Genet. 1995;4(5):807–12.

25. Aronson AE. Clinical voice disorders: an interdisciplinary approach. 3rd ed. New York: Thieme; 1990.

26. Ackermann H, Ziegler W. Cerebellar voice tremor: an acoustic analysis. J Neurol Neurosurg Psychiatry. 1991;54:74.

27. Chenery HJ, Ingram JCL, Murdoch BE. Perceptual analysis of the speech in ataxic dysarthria. Aust J Hum Comm Disord. 1991;18:19–28.

28. Murdoch BE. Disartria: uma abordagem fisiológica para avaliação e tratamento. São Paulo: Lovise; 2005.

29. Duffy JR. Motor speech disorders. Substrates, differential diagnosis, and management. St Louis: Mosby; 1995.

30. Theodoro D, Murdoch BE, Stokes PD, Chenery HJ. Hypernasality in dysarthric speakers following severe closed head injury: a perceptual and instrumental analysis. Brain Inj. 1993;7(1):59–69.

31. Kent RD, Kent JF, Duffy JR, Thomas JE, Weismer G, Stuntebeck S. Ataxic dysarthria. J Speech Lang Hear Res. 2000;43(5):1275–89.

32. Schalling E, Hammarberg B, Hartelius L. Perceptual and acoustic analysis of speech in individuals with spinocerebellar ataxia (SCA). Logoped Phoniatr Vocol. 2007;32(1):31–46.

33. Casper MA, Raphael LJ, Harris KS, Geibel JM. Speech prosody in cerebellar ataxia. Int J Lang Commun Disord. 2007;42(4):407–26.

34. Spencer KA, Slocomb DL. The neural basis of ataxic dysarthria. Cerebellum. 2007;6(1):58–65.

35. Portnoy RA, Aronson AE. Diadochokinetic syllable rate and regularity in normal and in spastic and ataxic dysarthric subjects. J Speech Hear Disord. 1982;47(3):324–8.

36. Padovani M, Behlau M, Gielow I. Análise da diadococinesia articulatória e laríngea em indivíduos com e sem transtornos neurológicos. Santos: Trabalho apresentado no XII Congresso Brasileiro de Fonoaudiologia; 2005.

37. Baken RJ. Clinical measurement of speech and voice. Boston: College-Hill; 1987. p. 445–52.

38. Coutinho P. Doença de Machado Joseph: Estudo Clínico. Porto: Patológico e Epidemiológico de uma Doença de Origem Portuguesa; 1993.

39. Ramió-Torrentà L, Gomez E, Genis D. Swallowing in degenerative ataxias. J Neurol. 2006;253:875–81.

40. Logemann JA. Evaluation and treatment of swallowing disorders. San Diego: College Hill; 1983. p. 249.

41. Costa, M. Deglutição e disfagia—anatomia—fisiologia—videofluoroscopia (conceitos básicos). XV "Encontro Tutorial e analítico das bases morfofuncionais e videofluoroscópica da dinâmica de deglutição normal e patológica". Material Institucional. ICB. Universidade Federal do Rio de Janeiro; 2005.

42. Aviv JE. The normal swallow. In: Carrau RL, Murry T, editors. Comprehensive management of swallowing disorders. San Diego: Plural Publishing; 2006.

43. Diaféria G, Pedroso J, Park SW, Haddad L, Haddad F, Barsottini O. Fiberoptic endoscopic evaluation of swallowing findings in patients with Machado-Joseph disease. Paper presented in the 20th International Congress of Parkinson's Disease and Movement Disorders MDS, Berlin, 2016.

Rehabilitation in Essential Tremor

6

Maria Eliza Freitas and Renato P. Munhoz

Introduction

Essential tremor (ET) is one of the most prevalent disorders in neurology, affecting 0.4–0.9 % in the general population of all ages, reaching even higher prevalence with advancing age, ranging from 4.6 to 6.3 % for individuals above 65 years old [1]. Although the term "benign ET" was historically used to describe it as a mono-symptomatic disorder with no pathological changes on brain tissue examination, it is not unusual to observe cases in which the progressive and potentially disabling nature of ET is evident, leading to significant disability and affecting quality of life with prominent interference with activities of daily living. In addition, there is heated debate about the validity and caveats of a series of recent studies highlighting the possible pathological changes in addition to a high prevalence of nonmotor symptoms and imaging abnormalities. Another recent development in the understanding of this field is the general concept that the entity as a single disease may not exist and what we refer to as ET is in fact the phenomenological expression of a series of different disorders [2, 3].

In spite of controversies and significant developments, treatment remains limited and includes pharmacotherapy, surgery and nonpharmacological therapy. The focus of this review is to discuss non-pharmacological therapies, mostly related to rehabilitation.

M.E. Freitas, M.D. • R.P. Munhoz, M.D., Ph.D. (✉)
Morton and Gloria Shulman Movement Disorders Centre and the Edmond J. Safra Program in Parkinson's Disease, Toronto Western Hospital, University of Toronto, Toronto, ON, Canada
e-mail: renato.munhoz@uhn.ca

© Springer International Publishing Switzerland 2017
H.F. Chien, O.G.P. Barsottini (eds.), *Movement Disorders Rehabilitation*,
DOI 10.1007/978-3-319-46062-8_6

Clinical Features of ET

The phenomenological hallmark of ET, as its designation suggests, is the postural and kinetic tremor of the upper extremities present in up to 95 % of cases. However, any body part can be affected, including more commonly the head (30 %), lower extremities (10–15 %), and voice (20 %), in the vast majority of cases in combination [4]. The two most consistent risk factors for ET are age and a family history of tremor. In spite of ≥50 % of the affected individuals presenting a positive family history, the objective identification of genes related to increased susceptibility and monozygotic forms of ET has been difficult [5]. Recent studies have linked LINGO1, FUS, and TENM4 genes with a higher risk of developing ET; however, further studies are needed to confirm their pathogenicity [6].

As mentioned above, in recent years, studies have shown that individuals with ET may develop nonmotor symptoms, such as cognitive deficits, depression, anxiety, balance disorder, hearing impairment, olfactory dysfunction, and sleep problems with a significant impact on quality of life [7]. Again, these topics and studies are currently a matter of heated debate among experts in the field.

The same observation is valid for pathological changes in ET. These findings in the central nervous system include a reduction in cerebellar Purkinje cells and restricted Lewy bodies in the locus ceruleus in a limited number of autopsied cases [8]. Brain imaging also shows changes in the cerebellum. A recent study using functional MRI and EEG showed an association between tremor and activity in the ipsilateral cerebellum and contralateral thalamus [9]. However, pathological and imaging changes are still a matter of controversy in the literature.

Pharmacological and Surgical Therapies

Pharmacological Approach

Oral pharmacotherapy in ET comprises different medications, including beta-blockers, anticonvulsants (primidone and topiramate), and benzodiazepines. Treatment may bring varying degrees of improvement in tremor severity in approximately 50 % of the patients, although this proportion diminishes as the disease progresses to more severe stages [10]. In general, treatment choice is based on the degree of psychological, social, and functional disability, and according to the general health status, as all pharmacological choices carry a significant risk of inducing adverse effects.

First-line therapy agents include propranolol and primidone. Propranolol is a nonselective β-adrenergic receptor antagonist and is the only pharmacotherapy approved through the US Food and Drug Administration (FDA). Initial doses of 20 mg twice a day are usually recommended (10 mg, twice a day in elderly patients). Doses can be titrated up to 60–320 mg/day. Common side effects are bradycardia and bronchospasm. Primidone is an anticonvulsant drug and the initial dose is 50 mg at bedtime (25 mg in elderly patients). Typical maintenance daily dose is

250–750 mg/day. The most frequent side effects are somnolence and dizziness. Second-line therapies include benzodiazepines (i.e., alprazolam), gabapentin, pregabalin, and topiramate.

Botulinum toxin type A (BTXA) has been proven to be effective in ET patients with tremors of the upper extremities [4]. Furthermore, BTXA is also effective in ET patients with head and voice tremors.

Essential tremor is classically marked by alcohol responsiveness. Ethanol improves tremor at relatively low levels, usually within 20 min for 3–5 h, sometimes followed by a rebound tremor augmentation [11]. Alcohol provides reduction in tremor amplitude, but not frequency. Given the significant improvement in tremors, alcohol addiction needs to be monitored in ET patients.

Surgical Approach

Deep brain stimulation (DBS) is the surgical treatment recommended for patients with disabling ETs. In 1997, the FDA approved DBS as a treatment for ET [12]. The ventrolateral thalamus and the posterior subthalamic area (PSA) are the typical targets for DBS in ET. Compared with unilateral implants, bilateral implants significantly reduce tremors; however, with a higher risk of side effects from stimulation (balance and posture). The effect is safe, with effects that are quite significant and long-lasting in most cases [13]. Thalamotomy is a surgical option that is equally as effective for refractory tremors in ET patients, but is limited because of an increased relative risk of adverse effects, especially with bilateral surgery.

Nonpharmacological Therapy and Rehabilitation

Although symptoms of ET may be controlled with medication or surgical interventions, it is of interest to explore and employ additional forms of therapy to assist with functionality. As already summarized, both medications and surgical interventions have several potential side effects and may not provide the best benefits in terms of overall motor function. Therefore, rehabilitation is in the pipeline not only for ET, but for most chronic neurological conditions. The interventions described below should typically be used in parallel with other forms of treatment or as the sole intervention.

Tremor

Resistance Training
The resistance training (RT) program is an exercise intervention consisting of sessions of biceps curl, wrist flexion, and wrist extension movements performed with both limbs with sets of repetitions. Exercises may be performed with loads.

A preliminary study reported that fine manual dexterity and upper limb strength were improved in ET patients after an RT program [14]. The findings of this preliminary study provided initial evidence that RT is worthy of further investigation as a therapy for improving functionality in ET patients.

A recent study investigated whether a generalized upper limb RT program improves manual dexterity and reduces force tremor in older individuals with ET [15]. Ten ET patients and 9 controls were recruited to participate in a 6-week program of upper-limb RT. A battery of manual dexterity and isometric force tremor assessments were performed before and after the RT to determine the benefits of the program. The 6-week, high-load, RT program produced strength increases in each limb for the ET and healthy older group. These changes in strength were associated with improvements in manual dexterity and tremor, particularly in the ET group. The least affected limb and the most affected limb exhibited similar improvements in functional assessments of manual dexterity, whereas reductions in force tremor amplitude following the RT program were restricted to the most affected limb of the ET group. These findings suggest that a generalized upper limb RT program has the potential to improve aspects of manual dexterity and reduce force tremor in older ET patients.

Inertial Loading

Inertial loading has been postulated to have an effect on the strength of motor unit training and the synergistic/competitive interaction between central and mechanical reflex tremor components in individuals with ET. A research study recruited 23 patients with ET and 22 controls and first defined the one-repetition maximum (1-RM) load, which is the maximal load that can be successfully lifted (wrist extensors) through the full range of motion [16]. Subsequently, the participants were asked to hold their hand in an outstretched position while supporting sub-maximal loads (no-load, 5, 15, and 25 % of 1-RM). Hand postural tremor and wrist extensor neuromuscular activity (electromyography [EMG]) were recorded. Results showed that inertial loading resulted in a reduction in postural tremor in all ET patients. The largest reduction in tremor amplitude occurred at between 5 and 15 % loads, which were associated with spectral separation of the mechanical reflex and central tremor components in a large number of ET subjects. Despite an increase in overall neuromuscular activity with inertial loading, EMG tremor spectral power did not increase with loading. The authors concluded that the effect of inertial loading on postural tremor amplitude appears to be mediated in large part by its effect on the interaction between the mechanical reflex and central tremor components.

Dexterity Training

Another technique that has been evaluated is exercise involving fine dexterity. A recent study evaluated the effect of a short-term dexterity training (DT) program on muscle tremor and the performance of hand precision tasks in patients with ET [17]. The study consisted of three testing sessions: baseline, after 4 weeks without any interventions (control), and after 4 weeks of a DT program carried out 3 times per week. Eight patients with ET were recruited and the training program consisted of

12 dexterity training sessions, each session comprising four tasks, involving both goal-directed manual movements and hand postural exercises. ET-specific quality of life questionnaires and postural and kinetic tremor assessments were performed. Results showed improvements in the performance of the two goal-directed tasks ($P<0.01$); however, postural and kinetic tremors did not change. The authors concluded that DT could be effective in increasing fine manual control during goal-directed movements, but no changes in tremor severity were seen. The authors also claimed that one limitation might be the short training program (4 weeks) and training programs taking place over a longer period of time may be of greater benefit.

Transcutaneous Electric Nerve Stimulation

Transcutaneous electrical nerve stimulation (TENS) is currently used for analgesia in a broad range of medical conditions, such as peripheral nerve lesions, angina, dysmenorrhea, labor and delivery, osteoarticular diseases, burns, and some types of postoperative pain [18]. Despite its widespread clinical use, the physiological mechanism of action is not known, stimulating parameters are subjective, electrode placement is empirical, and most of all, its effectiveness is a subject of controversy. Regardless of these uncertainties, the use of TENS has been reported to be effective in anecdotal reports of cases with certain movement disorders, including ET. Unfortunately, the only study performed using standard objective methodology in 5 patients with ET and 2 with peripheral tremor, did not reveal any significant improvement in the tremor scale scores after TENS, nor did it show any statistically significant difference in the amplitudes of the accelerometer tracings [19].

Massage

A recent study examined the influence of massage therapy on the severity of ET using an activity-based rating scale pre- and post-treatment [20]. The study consisted of five consecutive weekly sessions. The subject, a 63-year-old woman, indicated her hands and head to be the primary areas affected by ET. The treatment aim was to reduce sympathetic nervous system firing; therefore, the massage techniques implemented were based on relaxation. Methods included Swedish massage, hydrotherapy, myofascial release, diaphragmatic breathing, remedial exercise education and affirmative symptom management recommendations. Drawings of an Archimedes spiral for comparison pre- and post-treatment provided an objective, visual representation of tremor intensity affecting fine motor control. Goniometric measurements were taken to mark changes in cervical range of motion. Results revealed that tremor intensity decreased after each session, demonstrated by improved fine motor skills. The client also reported increased functionality in the cervical range of motion, which was documented during the first and last visits. The authors suggested that tremors in ET might be related to symptomatic activity and can be reduced by initiatives that encourage a parasympathetic response. Therefore, massage therapy would be a valuable method of treatment for ET. However, the study only examined 1 patient and tremor severity can present in an irregular pattern owing to subjective individual triggers. Further controlled research studies are required to lessen the variability between subjects and to validate these findings.

Gait

Essential tremor is marked by kinetic, postural, and intention tremors; however, many studies have suggested an underlying dysfunction of the cerebellum or cerebellar system causing gait and balance problems. Older age (>70 years) was consistently found to increase the risk of balance and gait disturbances in ET [21].

Louis et al. [22] studied the functional aspects of gait in patients with ET, placing their findings within the context of two other neurological disorders, Parkinson's disease and dystonia, and comparing them with age-matched controls. The authors administered the six-item Activities of Balance Confidence (ABC-6) Scale, which is a self-administered questionnaire that scores the level of confidence in performing different activities, such as standing on tiptoes to reach for an object, or walking outside on icy sidewalks, without losing balance or becoming unsteady. They also collected data on the number of falls and near-falls, and the use of walking aids in 422 participants (126 with ET, 77 with PD, 46 with dystonia, and 173 controls). Results showed that balance confidence was lowest in PD, intermediate in ET, and relatively preserved in dystonia compared with controls. The number of near-falls and falls followed a similar ordering. Use of canes, walkers, and wheelchairs was elevated in ET and even greater in PD. The authors concluded that lower balance confidence, increased number of falls, and a greater need for walking aids are variably features of patients with range of movement disorder compared with age-matched controls. Although most marked among PD patients, these issues affected ET patients and, to a small degree, some patients with dystonia.

A recent study compared timing control of gait in ET patients versus controls, and further assessed the association of these timing impairments with tremor severity among the ET patients [23]. One hundred and fifty-five ET patients and 60 age-matched controls underwent a comprehensive neurological assessment and gait analysis, which included walking at a criterion step frequency (cadence) with a metronome (timing production) and walking at a criterion step frequency after the metronome was turned off (timing reproduction). Outcomes of interest for both conditions were timing accuracy (measured by cadence error) and timing precision (measured by cadence variability). Results showed that cadence was lower in ET patients than in controls ($P<0.03$), whereas step time was similar for ET patients and controls. Accuracy (cadence error) and precision (cadence variability) were not different in ET patients compared with controls. Cranial tremor score was significantly associated with cadence (timing production condition, $P=0.003$, and timing reproduction condition, $P=0.0001$) and cadence error (timing production condition, $P=0.01$). Kinetic tremor and intention tremor scores were not associated with gait measures. The study concluded that ET patients do not demonstrate impairments in the timing of gait control compared with matched controls, in keeping with the hypothesis that the cerebellum might be important for timing the control of discrete rather than continuous movements.

It is well recognized that ET patients have gait and balance impairment [24]; however, most of the studies published on nonpharmacological approaches involve patients with PD, only revealing a gap in the literature in terms of treatment of ET gait disorders. Unmet needs in this field include randomized studies comparing ET patients and matched controls to assess the impact of physiotherapy and rehabilitation on gait and balance disorders in patients with ET.

References

1. Louis ED, Ferreira JJ. How common is the most common adult movement disorder? Update on the worldwide prevalence of essential tremor. Mov Disord. 2010;25(5):534–41.
2. Govert F, Deuschl G. Tremor entities and their classification: an update. Curr Opin Neurol. 2015;28(4):393–9.
3. Louis ED. Essential tremor: from bedside to bench and back to bedside. Curr Opin Neurol. 2014;27(4):461–7.
4. Chunling W, Zheng X. Review on clinical update of essential tremor. Neurol Sci. 2016;37(4):495–502.
5. Tio M, Tan E-K. Genetics of essential tremor. Parkinsonism Relat Disord. 2016;22 Suppl 1:S176–8.
6. Agúndez JA, Jiménez-Jimenez FJ, Alonso-Navarro H, García-Martín E. The potential of LINGO-1 as a therapeutic target for essential tremor. Expert Opin Ther Targets. 2015;19(8):1139–48.
7. Musacchio T, Purrer V, Papagianni A, Fleischer A, Mackenrodt D, Malsch C, et al. Non-motor symptoms of essential tremor are independent of tremor severity and have an impact on quality of life. Tremor Other Hyperkinet Mov (N Y). 2016;6:361.
8. Shill HA, Adler CH, Beach TG. Pathology in essential tremor. Parkinsonism Relat Disord. 2012;18:S135–7.
9. Contarino MF, Groot PFC, van der Meer JN, Bour LJ, Speelman JD, Nederveen AJ, et al. Is there a role for combined EMG-fMRI in exploring the pathophysiology of essential tremor and improving functional neurosurgery? PLoS One. 2012;7(10), e46234.
10. Broccard FD, Mullen T, Chi YM, Peterson D, Iversen JR, Arnold M, et al. Closed-loop brain-machine-body interfaces for noninvasive rehabilitation of movement disorders. Ann Biomed Eng. 2014;42(8):1573–93.
11. Ondo W. Essential tremor: what we can learn from current pharmacotherapy. Tremor Other Hyperkinet Mov (N Y). 2016;6:356.
12. Munhoz RP, Picillo M, Fox SH, Bruno V, Panisset M, Honey CR, Fasano A. Eligibility criteria for deep brain stimulation in Parkinson's disease, tremor, and dystonia. Can J Neurol Sci. 2016;3:1–10.
13. Baizabal-Carvallo JF, Kagnoff MN. The safety and efficacy of thalamic deep brain stimulation in essential tremor: 10 years and beyond. J Neurol. 2014;85(5):567–72.
14. Sequeira G, Keogh JW, Kavanagh JJ. Resistance training can improve fine manual dexterity in essential tremor patients: a preliminary study. Arch Phys Med Rehabil. 2012;93(8):1466–8.
15. Kavanagh JJ, Wedderburn-Bisshop J, Keogh JWL. Resistance training reduces force tremor and improves manual dexterity in older individuals with essential tremor. J Mot Behav. 2016;48(1):20–30.
16. Héroux ME, Pari G, Norman KE. The effect of inertial loading on wrist postural tremor in essential tremor. Clin Neurophysiol. 2009;120(5):1020–9.
17. Budini F, Lowery MM, Hutchinson M, Bradley D, Conroy L, De Vito G. Dexterity training improves manual precision in patients affected by essential tremor. Arch Phys Med Rehabil. 2014;95(4):705–10.
18. Carroll D, Moore RA, McQuay HJ, Fairman F, Leijon G. Transcutaneous electrical nerve stimulation for chronic pain. Cochrane Database Syst Rev. 2001;3, CD003222.
19. Munhoz RP, Hanajima R, Ashby P, Lang AE. Acute effect of transcutaneous electrical nerve stimulation on tremor. Mov Disord. 2003;18(2):191–4.

20. Riou N. Massage therapy for essential tremor: quieting the mind. J Bodyw Mov Ther. 2013;17(4):488–94.
21. Rao AK, Gillman A, Louis ED. Quantitative gait analysis in essential tremor reveals impairments that are maintained into advanced age. Gait Posture. 2011;34(1):65–70.
22. Louis ED, Rao AK. Functional aspects of gait in essential tremor: a comparison with age-matched Parkinson's disease cases dystonia cases and controls. Tremor Other Hyperkinet Mov (N Y). 2015;5:5–308. Center for Research and Digital Scholarship, Columbia University.
23. Rao AK, Louis ED. Timing control of gait: a study of essential tremor patients vs. age-matched controls. Cerebellum Ataxias. 2016;3(1):5.
24. Arkadir D, Louis ED. The balance and gait disorder of essential tremor: what does this mean for patients? Ther Adv Neurol Disord. 2013;6(4):229–36.

Rehabilitation in Chorea

7

Débora Maia and Francisco Cardoso

Introduction

The term "chorea" derives from the Greek word "choreia," which means dance, and is used to define a syndrome characterized by involuntary movements that are brief, abrupt, unpredictable and nonrhythmic, resulting from a continuous flow of random muscle contractions.

Causes of chorea may be categorized by etiology into genetic and acquired, with significant implications for management and prognosis. Regardless of its cause (Table 7.1) [1], the two types has similar common features and many patients present with functional disability in addition to dysphagia, dysarthria, and impairment of gait and balance. The purpose of rehabilitation is to tackle these functional impairments .

The aim of this chapter is to provide an overview of rehabilitation in the most frequent forms of non-Huntington's chorea. It is important to emphasize that most of the information provided herein is based on the personal experience of the authors as there is a paucity of data in the field. The strategy we have followed in the chapter is to start with a succinct description of general aspects of each specific cause of chorea, followed by discussion of rehabilitation.

D. Maia, M.D., M.Sc. • F. Cardoso, M.D., Ph.D., F.A.A.N. (✉)
Movement Disorders Unit, Neurology Service, The Federal University
of Minas Gerais, Belo Horizonte, MG, Brazil
e-mail: cardosofe@terra.com.br

© Springer International Publishing Switzerland 2017
H.F. Chien, O.G.P. Barsottini (eds.), *Movement Disorders Rehabilitation*,
DOI 10.1007/978-3-319-46062-8_7

Table 7.1 Causes of chorea (adapted with permission from Cardoso [1])

Inherited	Autosomal dominant	HD
		HDL-1, HDL-2, HDL-4/SCA17
		Spinocerebellar ataxias (SCA1, SCA2, SCA3, SCA7, SCA8, SCA14, SCA17, SCA27 (van Gaalen 2011)
		DRPLA
		Neuroferritinopathy
		BHC
		ADCY5-related dyskinesia
		C9ORF72
		GLUT1 deficiency
		POLG (may be autosomal dominant or recessive)
		PRRT2 mutations
	Autosomal recessive	Chorea-acanthocytosis
		Friedreich's ataxia
		Wilson's disease
		AOA 1 and 2
		PKAN
		Ataxia–telangiectasia
		POLG
		Inborn errors of metabolism (e.g., phenylketonuria, glutaric acidemia type I, methylglutaconic aciduria type III)
	X-linked recessive	McLeod neuro-acanthocytosis
		Lesch–Nyhan syndrome
		Rett syndrome
	Mitochondrial	Leigh syndrome
		Lactic acidosis and stroke-like episodes (MELAS)
		Leber hereditary optic neuropathy (Morimoto 2004)
Acquired	Vascular/hypoxic-ischemic injury	Stroke
		Post-pump chorea
		Perinatal hypoxic injury
		Polycythemia vera
	Immune-mediated	Sydenham's chorea
		Systemic lupus erythematosus, Sjögren's syndrome
		Antiphospholipid antibody syndrome
		Chorea gravidarum
		Oral contraceptives
		Immune encephalopathies (anti-LGI1, CASPR2 and NMDA receptor antibodies)
		Celiac disease
	Metabolic disorders	Nonketotic hyperglycemia
		Hyperthyroidism
		Hypoparathyroidism
		Uremia
	Paraneoplastic	Renal, small cell, lung, breast, Hodgkin's lymphoma, non-Hodgkin's lymphoma
	Infective	HIV
		Syphilis
		Mycoplasma
		Legionella
		Varicella
		Herpes simplex
	Drugs/toxins	Mercury
		Cocaine
		Amphetamines
Idiopathic		

Genetic Chorea

Neuro-acanthocytosis

Neuro-acanthocytosis is a genetically and phenotypically heterogeneous group of disorders that includes chorea-acanthocytosis and McLeod syndrome [2]. Chorea-acanthocytosis is a rare autosomal recessive disorder caused by mutations in the VPS13A gene on chromosome 9q21, which encodes the protein chorein. The disease typically presents in adulthood, with a mean age of 30 years, and rarely before the age of 20 or after the age of 50 years. Chorea acanthocytosis is relentlessly progressive, and sufferers may develop significant disability within a few years [3].

Affected individuals develop a mixed movement disorder, typically involving chorea and dystonia, and occasionally Parkinsonism later in the course of the disease, in addition to other neurological features such as seizures, neuropathy, and myopathy [2, 4]. The chorea in chorea-acanthocytosis is generalized, affecting the limbs, face, and trunk, and often interferes with ambulation, causing frequent falls. Co-existing dystonia is often present. There may be prominent oral involvement, and the presence of feeding-related tongue dystonia or self-mutilatory mouth movements, often appearing early in the course of the disease, provide a useful clue to the diagnosis [5]. Head drop and axial extension have also been reported to be characteristic features in advanced disease [6]. Cognitive and behavioral disturbances are seen in the majority of affected individuals [2] and neuropsychiatric symptoms may precede the onset of the movement disorder [7].

McLeod neuro-acanthocytosis syndrome is an X-linked recessive disorder, caused by mutations in the XK gene located at Xp21.1, which encodes an antigen of the Kell blood group [7]. Affected males manifest a progressive chorea syndrome, in addition to cognitive and behavioral disturbances. Reports of heterozygous females manifesting chorea and cognitive disturbance have also been identified [2]. Similar to chorea-acanthocytosis, seizures and subclinical neuromuscular disease are also present. The chorea is generalized and often interferes with ambulation with frequent falls. Hematologically, the McLeod blood group phenotype is characterized by absent expression of the Kx erythrocyte antigen and reduced expression of the Kell blood group antigen, leading to acanthocytosis and compensated hemolysis. In contrast to those with chorea-acanthocytosis, affected individuals may also develop dilated cardiomyopathy and arrhythmias, with a risk of sudden cardiac death.

Wilson's Disease

Wilson's disease is an autosomal recessive disorder caused by mutations in the ATP7B gene on chromosome 13q14.3, which encodes for a copper transporting P-type transmembrane ATPase [8]. The age at onset ranges from early childhood to the sixth decade of life, with a mean age of onset between 15 and 21 years. The majority of affected individuals are dysarthric, with varying spastic, ataxic, hypokinetic, and dystonic components to their speech. Neurological Wilson's disease may present with dystonia, tremor or parkinsonism, or a combination of movement disorders. Chorea has been reported in 6–16% of cases, and tends to accompany other neurological manifestations.

Benign Hereditary Chorea

Benign hereditary chorea (BHC) is classically caused by autosomal dominant mutations in the *NKX2.1* (TITF1) gene, located on the long arm of chromosome 14 [9]. There is a slight female preponderance, with a male to female ratio of 0.70 [10]. Usually, affected individuals develop generalized chorea with onset during early childhood, with a median age of 2.5–3 years, although onset from infancy to late childhood and adolescence has also been described [11]. Chorea is worsened with stress, and improves during sleep. There is often a history of decreased muscle in the first year of life, in addition to delayed motor milestones, particularly with walking. The chorea tends to improve up until puberty or early adulthood, before stabilizing during adulthood [10]. Infrequently, there may be a complete resolution of chorea. Associated movement disorders have also been described, including myoclonus, dystonia, tics, and drop attacks. In some cases, as chorea improves with age, myoclonus becomes the main disabling symptom in adulthood. Dysarthria has also been reported [12]. Nonmotor features are additionally associated with BHC, and include learning difficulties, which were observed in 20 out of 28 individuals in one series [10], and attention deficit hyperactivity disorder (ADHD). Cerebral imaging in BHC is typically normal.

The mutation in ADCY5, the gene described in 2001 and linked to familial dyskinesia with facial myokymia, has been reported in patients with a phenotype of BHC. In general, patients present with hyperkinetic movements, mainly chorea and dystonia, but also other forms of dyskinesia. Quite often, they have preserved cognition and no other major neurological features. In contrast to BHC cases secondary to NKX2-1 mutations, patients with ADCY5 mutation may show significant progression of symptoms until adulthood. Facial myokymia, cardiac heart failure, more prominent dystonic posturing, and even cognitive decline may occur in ADCY5-related disorder [13].

C9orf72 Disease

C9orf72 disease is an autosomal dominant condition caused by an expanded hexanucleotide repeat in the C9orf72 gene. This was originally described in a Finnish and a European cohort [14] and in a family of Irish descent [15] with familial frontotemporal lobar degeneration (FTLD) and amyotrophic lateral sclerosis (ALS). This is considered the most common genetic cause of FTLD-ALSC9orf72 disease is an autosomal dominant condition caused by an expanded hexanucleotide repeat in the C9orf72 gene. This was originally described in a Finnish and European cohort

[14] and a family of Irish descent [15] with familial frontotemporal lobar degeneration (FTLD) and amyotrophic lateral sclerosis (ALS). This is considered the most common genetic cause of FTLD-ALS.

In a large Huntington's disease (HD) phenocopy cohort [16], the mean age of onset was 42.7 years. Affected individuals manifested chorea, dystonia, myoclonus, tremor, and parkinsonism. Upper motor neuron signs were also present in some affected individuals. Executive dysfunction was common, and psychiatric and behavioral problems tended to occur early. No clear differences in the size of the expanded hexanucleotide repeat have been identified to account for the varied phenotypic presentations of C9orf72 disease. Incomplete penetrance has been described and generalized atrophy may be observed on MRI.

DRPLA

An autosomal dominant disorder, DRPLA is caused by an expanded CAG repeat in the *DRPLA* gene (atrophin 1) located on chromosome 12p13.31 [17]. Anticipation is a feature of DRPLA, with intergenerational expansion typically associated with paternal transmission. The normal repeat range is 8–25, whereas the reported range in affected individuals is from 49 to 88 [18]. DRPLA occurs more commonly in Japan, where the prevalence is estimated to be 0.2–07 per 100,000 [19]. It is very rare in other ethnic populations.

The age at onset ranges from the first to the seventh decade [17]. The clinical features of DRPLA vary according to the age of onset, with striking differences between the juvenile and adult-onset forms. The juvenile form of the disease, with age at onset before 20 years, is characterized by a progressive myoclonus epilepsy phenotype, with myoclonus, epilepsy, and mental retardation. In contrast, adult-onset DRPLA progresses more slowly, with varying degrees of ataxia, choreoathetosis, and subcortical dementia. Epilepsy and myoclonus do not tend to occur.

Nongenetic Chorea

Nongenetic forms of chorea are a group of heterogeneous conditions that may include chorea at any moment during the course of the disease. Table 7.1 also shows a comprehensive list of causes of acquired chorea. Because of their frequency, the most important etiologies are vascular and immunological disorders.

Cerebrovascular disease is the most common cause of nongenetic chorea in adults, accounting for 50% of cases [20]. However, chorea is an unusual complication of acute vascular lesions, seen in less than 1% of patients with acute stroke. Vascular hemichorea or hemiballism (severe chorea) is usually related to ischemic or hemorrhagic lesions of the basal ganglia and adjacent white matter in the territory of the middle or the posterior cerebral arteries. Although spontaneous remission is the rule, in a few patients, the movement disorder may persist and treatment with antichoreic drugs, such as neuroleptics or dopamine depleters, may be necessary in the acute phase.

Sydenham's chorea (SC) is the most common form of autoimmune chorea. In fact, it is the most common cause of acute chorea in children worldwide. SC is a major feature of acute rheumatic fever, an autoimmune disease related to previous infection with group A beta-hemolytic *Streptococcus* [21]. Clinically, SC is characterized by a combination of chorea, other movement disorders, behavioral abnormalities, difficulties in verbal fluency and in verbal comprehension, and cognitive changes [22–24]. Oliveira et al. [25] demonstrated that patients with acute SC have an impairment of modulation of the voice and longer duration of emission of sentences, resulting in a monotone and slow speech. This pattern is similar to that described in other basal ganglia illnesses, such as Parkinson's disease and Huntington's disease.

Other immunological causes of chorea are systemic lupus erythematosus (SLE), primary antiphospholipid antibody syndrome, vasculitis, and paraneoplastic syndromes. SLE and antiphospholipid antibody syndrome are classically described as the prototypes of autoimmune chorea [26]. However, several reports show that chorea is seen in no more than 1% to 2% of large series of patients with these conditions [27–29]. Autoimmune chorea has rarely been reported in the context of paraneoplastic syndromes associated with CV2/CRMP5 antibodies in patients with small-cell lung carcinoma or malignant thymoma [30].

Rehabilitation

Dysarthria

Dysarthria is often a disabling problem in genetic chorea and less so in individuals with vascular chorea. In these cases speech therapy is of benefit. Unfortunately, in degenerative chorea there is a relentless progression with patients with advanced disease commonly becoming anarthric. In immunological and other forms of acquired chorea, dysarthria is usually mild and self-limited and does not require specific therapeutic measures.

Dysphagia

Dysphagia is a significant problem in neuro-acanthocytosis, Wilson's disease, phenocopies of HD, and other degenerative causes of non-HD chorea. In the early stages of these conditions, speech therapy may benefit patients with dysphagia [2]. Clinical experience suggests that these measures might decrease the likelihood of aspiration pneumonia, but published data to support this assumption are lacking. Unfortunately, given the progressive nature of these conditions, there is a relentless worsening of dysphagia, with many patients becoming unable to swallow. In these circumstances, there is an indication for the use of gastrostomy. Despite the widespread belief that this procedure prevents aspiration pneumonia, there is inconclusive evidence to support this conclusion.

A task-specific dystonia with protrusion of the tongue pushing food out of the mouth is a cause of quite specific chewing and swallowing problems in up to 50% of patients with chorea-acanthocytosis. In these cases, the use of a mechanical device such a stick to reduce biting and tooth-grinding can be helpful and avoid teeth having to be removed [3]. Botulinum toxin injections into the genioglossus may reduce tongue protrusion and improve feeding and speech as well [3]. In patients with bruxism, botulinum toxin in the masseter and temporal muscles can also be helpful.

Malnutrition

Chorea patients with severe dysphagia may develop malnutrition. It is therefore necessary to carefully monitor the nutritional status of these individuals and nutritionists should be part of the multidisciplinary team caring for these patients. As already discussed in the section on dysphagia, at end-stage degenerative chorea, many patients require gastrostomy to maintain proper nutrition and possibly reduce the risk of aspiration pneumonia.

Gait Disturbance and Postural Instability

In 2005, Danek and Walker described the importance of physical therapy in improving gait and balance in patients with neuro-acanthocytosis. However, not only in this condition but also in chorea in general, there are no specific protocols. As in other progressive disorders, physiotherapy is frequently directed toward maintaining or retraining personal independence: reach to grasp movement, bed mobility, transfers, and walking. When mobility becomes further compromised, assistive devices for walking may become necessary. Unfortunately, in degenerative conditions associated with chorea, there is a steady and relentless progression, with patients becoming wheelchair bound and, later in the course of the disease, confined to bed.

There are no specific data in the literature about the role of physical therapy in immunological chorea. As a matter of fact, in the experience of the authors, with the exception of bilateral vascular hemiballism–hemichorea and chorea paralytica, a rare form of SC, physical therapy is not necessary in acquired chorea. Of note, physiotherapy is required to avoid spasticity and improve gait and balance in patients with hemiparesis in vascular chorea.

Conclusion

Because of the rarity of these conditions, all reports of therapies are anecdotal, and no controlled clinical trials have been performed. Treatment for most of the symptoms of nongenetic chorea syndromes is based upon empirical evidence from patients with other conditions such as Huntington's disease. There are, however, some reports that suggest that a multi-disciplinary approach might improve functional disturbances.

References

1. Cardoso F. Huntington disease and other choreas. Neurol Clin. 2009;27:719–36.
2. Danek A, Walker RH. Neuroacanthocytosis. Curr Opin Neurol. 2005;18(4):386–92.
3. Walker R. Management of neuroacanthocytosis syndromes. Tremor Other Hyperkinet Mov. 2015;5:346.
4. Peppard RF, Lu CS, Chu NS, Teal P, Martin WR, Calne DB. Parkinsonism with neuroacanthocytosis. Can J Neurol Sci. 1990;17(3):298–301.
5. Bader B, Walker RH, Vogel M, Prosiegel M, McIntosh J, Danek A. Tongue protrusion and feeding dystonia: a hallmark of chorea-acanthocytosis. Mov Disord. 2010;25(1):127–9.
6. Schneider SA, Lang AE, Moro E, Bader B, Danek A, Bhatia KP. Characteristic head drops and axial extension in advanced chorea-acanthocytosis. Mov Disord. 2010;25(10):1487–91.
7. Walker RH, Jung HH, Dobson-Stone C, Rampoldi L, Sano A, Tison F, Danek A. Neurologic phenotypes associated with acanthocytosis. Neurology. 2007;68(2):92–8.
8. Lorincz MT. Neurologic Wilson's disease. Ann N Y Acad Sci. 2010;1184:173–87.
9. Breedveld GJ, van Dongen JW, Danesino C, et al. Mutations in TITF-1 are associated with benign hereditary chorea. Hum Mol Genet. 2002;11:971–9.
10. Gras D, Jonard L, Roze E, Chantot-Bastaraud S, Koht J, Motte J, Rodriguez D, Louha M, Caubel I, Kemlin I, Lion-François L, Goizet C, Guillot L, Moutard ML, Epaud R, Héron B, Charles P, Tallot M, Camuzat A, Durr A, Polak M, Devos D, Sanlaville D, Vuillaume I, Billette de Villemeur T, Vidailhet M, Doummar D. Benign hereditary chorea: phenotype, prognosis, therapeutic outcome and long term follow-up in a large series with new mutations in the TITF1/NKX2-1 gene. J Neurol Neurosurg Psychiatry. 2012;83(10):956–62.
11. Kleiner-Fisman G, Lang AE. Benign hereditary chorea revisited: a journey to understanding. Mov Disord. 2007;22(16):2297–305. quiz 2452.
12. Asmus F, Horber V, Pohlenz J, Schwabe D, Zimprich A, Munz M, Schöning M, Gasser T. A novel TITF-1 mutation causes benign hereditary chorea with response to levodopa. Neurology. 2005;64(11):1952–4.
13. Mencacci NE, Erro R, Wiethoff S, et al. ADCY5 mutations are another cause of benign hereditary chorea. Neurology. 2015;85:80–8.
14. Renton AE, Majounie E, Waite A, et al. A hexanucleotide repeat expansion in C9ORF72 is the cause of chromosome 9p21-linked ALS-FTD. Neuron. 2011;72(2):257–68.
15. Boxer AL, Mackenzie IR, Boeve BF, Baker M, Seeley WW, Crook R, Feldman H, Hsiung GY, Rutherford N, Laluz V, Whitwell J, Foti D, McDade E, Molano J, Karydas A, Wojtas A, Goldman J, Mirsky J, Sengdy P, Dearmond S, Miller BL, Rademakers R. Clinical, neuroimaging and neuropathological features of a new chromosome 9p-linked FTD-ALS family. J Neurol Neurosurg Psychiatry. 2011;82(2):196–203.
16. Hensman Moss DJ, Poulter M, Beck J, Hehir J, Polke JM, Campbell T, Adamson G, Mudanohwo E, McColgan P, Haworth A, Wild EJ, Sweeney MG, Houlden H, Mead S, Tabrizi SJ. C9orf72 expansions are the most common genetic cause of Huntington disease phenocopies. Neurology. 2014;82(4):292–9.
17. Koide R, Ikeuchi T, Onodera O, Tanaka H, Igarashi S, Endo K, Takahashi H, Kondo R, Ishikawa A, Hayashi T, et al. Unstable expansion of CAG repeat in hereditary dentatorubral-pallidoluysian atrophy (DRPLA). Nat Genet. 1994;6(1):9–13.
18. Gövert F, Schneider SA. Huntington's disease and Huntington's disease-like syndromes: an overview. Curr Opin Neurol. 2013;26(4):420–7.
19. Le Ber I, Camuzat A, Castelnovo G, Azulay JP, Genton P, Gastaut JL, Broglin D, Labauge P, Brice A, Durr A. Prevalence of dentatorubral-pallidoluysian atrophy in a large series of white patients with cerebellar ataxia. Arch Neurol. 2003;60(8):1097–9.
20. Piccolo I, Defanti CA, Soliveri P, et al. Cause and course in a series of patients with sporadic chorea. J Neurol. 2003;250:429–35.
21. Cardoso F, Seppi K, Mair KJ, et al. Seminar on choreas. Lancet Neurol. 2006;5:589–6021.
22. Maia DP, Teixeira Jr AL, Cunningham MCQ, Cardoso F. Obsessive compulsive behavior, hyperactivity and attention deficit disorder in Sydenham chorea. Neurology. 2005;64:1799–801.

23. Harsányi E, Moreira J, Kummer A, et al. Language impairment in adolescents with sydenham chorea. Pediatr Neurol. 2015;53(5):412–16.
24. Beato R, Maia DP, Teixeira Jr AL, Cardoso F. Executive functioning in adult patients with Sydenham's chorea. Mov Disord. 2010;27(7):853–7.
25. Oliveira PM, Cardoso F, Maia DP, et al. Acoustic analysis of prosody in Sydenham's chorea. Arq Neuropsiquiatr. 2010;68(5):744–8.
26. Quinn N, Schrag A. Huntington's disease and other choreas. J Neurol. 1998;245:709–16.
27. Asherson RA, Cervera R. The antiphospholipid syndrome: multiple faces beyond the classical presentation. Autoimmun Rev. 2003;2(3):140–51. 128.
28. Avcin T, Benseler SM, Tyrrell PN, et al. A followup study of antiphospholipid antibodies and associated neuropsychiatric manifestations in 137 children with systemic lupus erythematosus. Arthritis Rheum. 2008;59(2):206–13.
29. Maciel ROH, Ferreira GA, Akemy B, Cardoso F. Executive dysfunction, obsessive-compulsive symptoms, and attention deficit and hyperactivity disorder in systemic lupus erythematosus: evidence for basal ganglia dysfunction? J Neurol Sci. 2016;360:94–7.
30. Honnorat J, Cartalat-Carel S, Ricard D, et al. Onco-neural antibodies and tumor type determine survival and neurological symptoms in paraneoplastic neurological syndromes with Hu or CV2/CRMP5 antibodies. J Neurol Neurosurg Psychiatry. 2009;80(4):412–16.

Huntington's Disease

8

Monica Santoro Haddad, Tamine Teixeira da Costa Capato, and Mariana Jardim Azambuja

Introduction

Huntington's disease (HD) is a genetic neurodegenerative disease with autosomal dominant inheritance characterized by chorea, cognitive, and behavioral impairments [1]. HD is caused by an expanded CAG trinucleotide repeat in the *HTT* gene [2]. Although chorea is the main type of involuntary movement and usually presents during any phase of the disease, other motor impairments appear, such as dystonia, bradykinesia, rigidity, and balance disturbances [3]. The general aspect of the HD gait is the enlarged basis with balance and movements up and down, which are responsible for causing frequent falls in 60 % of the patients [4]. HD-related cognitive deficits include processing speed, set-switching, sequencing, and distractibility, suggesting that the basal ganglia might play a role in many cognitive functions traditionally attributed to the frontal cortex [5].

Many pharmacological therapies have been evaluated; however, positive pharmacological results are still scanty; thus few treatment options are available [6, 7]. A few studies attempted to address the question as to which aspects of motor

M.S. Haddad, M.D., M.Sc. (✉)
Department of Neurology, Hospital das Clinicas da Faculdade de Medicina da Universidade São Paulo, São Paulo, Brazil
e-mail: haddad.monica@yahoo.com.br; mshaddad@uol.com.br

T.T. da Costa Capato, P.T., M.Sc.
Department of Physical Therapy, Hospital das Clínicas da Faculdade de Medicina da Universidade de São Paulo, São Paulo, Brazil
e-mail: taminec@yahoo.com.br

M.J. Azambuja, S.L.P., M.Sc.
Department of Neurology, Hospital das Clinicas da Faculdade de Medicina da Universidade de São Paulo, São Paulo, Brazil
e-mail: marianaazambuja@hotmail.com.br

© Springer International Publishing Switzerland 2017
H.F. Chien, O.G.P. Barsottini (eds.), *Movement Disorders Rehabilitation*,
DOI 10.1007/978-3-319-46062-8_8

function improve when chorea is reduced with tetrabenazine or other antichoreic treatments [8]. Studies suggest that globus pallidus internus (GPi) deep brain stimulation (DBS) might be a potential therapeutic option in patients with refractory chorea, but few cases with long-term effects have been reported in the literature [9–11].

Death occurs after 15–20 years of the disease, usually because of trauma related to falls or infections related to dysphagia. Therefore, physical therapy and speech therapy are extremely important in avoiding these events.

This chapter reviews the main physical and speech therapy strategies that can improve quality of life of HD patients.

Physical Therapy

Even with the ideal medical and surgical treatment, HD patients still present problems with functional activities, gait and balance. Nevertheless, there are some suggestions that physiotherapy treatment might improve functional disturbances of the basal ganglia motor circuit. However, the mechanisms by which improvement occurs remain unexplained.

Main Goals of Physical Therapy

The main goals of physical therapy targeting HD can be divided into four different stages: pre-manifest, early stage, mid stage, and late stage.

Pre-manifest Stage

A person who has an unfavorable genetic test for the HD, but has not yet developed any clinical signs of HD is considered to be pre-manifest. Mild gait changes can be observed in pre-manifest individuals, including decreased gait velocity and stride length; increased double support time; and increased variability in stride length and step time compared with controls [12]. In a multicenter, prospective, observational study involving a total of eight sites, test measures of functional abilities and physical impairments were proposed in 81 people with pre-manifest and manifest HD. The preliminary results showed that specific measures may be appropriate for HD, and the tools may be useful to assessing individuals in the pre-manifest stage [13].

Even in the absence of any specific motor impairment limitation, the patients should be encouraged to undergo a specific evaluation with a physiotherapist specializing in movement disorders, and test the influence of cognitive issues on functional activities. All these physical interventions may include support the maintenance of an independent exercise program; however, the evidence is not strong and little is known about the dosage, frequency, and intensity at that stage.

Early Stage

At the early stage, there may be progression of cognitive deficits such as memory, planning, problem-solving, organizing, new learning, and attention. A mild postural instability and falls may occur in early and mid-stages of HD, and the mean incidence is approximately 58–60 %. The patients cannot report the numbers of falls exactly and the circumstances under which these falls occurred were due to the progression of cognitive impairments [4]. The balance impairments may be multifactorial such as the correct sequencing of postural responses, delays in initiation, and prolonged anticipatory postural adjustments [14], deficits in adapting the postural response to change task demands and environment and response to chorea, increased postural sway, impaired cognitive function and behavior, and reduced ability to maintain postural stability during dual tasks [4].

Altered musculoskeletal alignment, which may be associated with chorea and dystonia, disorders of the integration of sensory information, including dependence on proprioceptive cues rather than on visual cues. Lower-limb muscle weakness and reduced activity [15] are other factors. The side effects of some medications and environmental hazards may also contribute to the high incidence of falls [16].

Individuals with HD have been found to have a reduction in the quality of functional manual activities caused by chorea, bradykinesia, and difficulties in movement sequencing [17].

Gait impairments could be marked by a gait bradykinesia, the disorder of locomotor timing demonstrated by increased difficulty in the ability to regulate cadence and an increased variability of stepping rates. The timing disorder in HD may be the result of a dysfunction of the basal ganglia cueing mechanism that signals the supplementary motor areas to prepare the next movement in the sequence [18].

The slower stepping response time (STR) in HD may become slower gait, prolonged reaction time, and slower movement time of the upper extremity, and a longer reaction time and reduction in speed of the first step of ambulation in people with HD are consistent with bradykinesia being a feature of HD. In an investigation, the authors showed that deficits in SRT were associated with impairments on clinical measures of balance, mobility, and motor performance, including a subjective measure related to balance and confidence. The correlation suggested that in people with HD, slower response times might be associated with lower balance confidence during performance of common daily activities. Good correlations were found between SRT and clinical measures, such as timed up & go (TUG) and tandem walk tests, highlighting associations between SRT and gait-related performance measures. The slower SRT was associated with poorer performance on the TUG and the tandem walk tests. The results showed that SRT may be a valid and objective marker of disease progression [19].

The assessment of motor functions may be required; thus, in some studies evaluation is performed using a specific test proposed by the Guideline for Huntington's Disease [20] and others showed the importance of determining the efficacy of minimal detectable changes on measures before and after physical therapy interventions [21].

This evaluation should be carried out by a physical therapist specialized in neurology and movement disorders. This guideline can provide a general framework for physical therapy intervention for impairments that can have an impact on the functional activity and life participation of people with HD [20].

Gait retraining strategies for people with HD, therefore, need to target disorders of both footstep timing and amplitude [18]. There were a few exercise protocols aimed at people with HD. They suggest some strategies for training gait [22], functional activities [23, 24], and multi-sensory stimulation [25]. There are no specific balance protocols for HD; thus, we suggest the Parkinson's disease protocols, because they may be very useful for implementing the dosage, frequency, and intensity of the physical therapy sessions [26].

Aerobic exercises (walking—treadmill and over-ground, jogging, swimming, and stationary bicycling) are recommended in a frequency of 3–5 times a week, in an intensity of 65–85 % of the maximal heart rate. Exergaming, Yoga, Pilates, Tai Chi, and relaxation are also suggested [20].

Exercise adherence in this population decreases after professional supervision stops and patients no longer receive external support or feedback about their progress [17, 27]. There is clearly a need to develop methods that facilitate patients and caregivers engagement in and adherence to an exercise program.

The benefits of regular physical activity for people with HD are widely recognized. Although regular and sustained physical activity has the potential to benefit patients with neurodegenerative conditions such as HD, there are a number of disease-specific factors that make it particularly challenging to establish regular exercise in this population. For that reason, it is important to support engagement in physical activity in people with Huntington's disease with a study protocol for a randomized controlled feasibility trial [28].

Mid Stage

During the mid-stage of HD, involuntary movements such as chorea increase, dystonic postures (e.g., torticollis, opisthotonus, and arching of the feet) may be present and voluntary motor tasks may become increasingly difficult. People have balance and gait deficits, including increased variability in gait parameters (e.g., stride time and length, double support time) [12], that result in frequent falls [15]. Contributing factors may include bradykinesia of gait, stride variability, and chorea in addition to cognitive and behavioral issues [4]. People may also frequently drop objects that they are holding in their hands because of motor impersistence. Motor skill learning is also often impaired at this stage, resulting in difficulties learning new tasks or sequences [29].

The chorea or hypokinesia rigidity are characteristics that are independent predictors of both cognitive and general functioning, with choreatic patients functioning significantly better. The hypokinetic HD subtypes are associated with poorer functioning than the hyperkinetic. It is possible that choreatic subjects are falsely assigned to the hypokinetic rigid group because of medication-induced hypokinesia [30].

As the disease progresses, physiotherapy is frequently directed toward maintaining or retraining the reach to grasp movement, bed mobility, transfers, and walking. When mobility becomes further compromised, wheelchair prescription and training in wheelchair use may become a priority. In a systematic review, the overall aim of physical therapy in the mild stage was to facilitate independence in activities of daily life and optimize participation in family, work, and leisure. These aims may be achieved through an education, specific advice on safety and risk management, modification of activities or environments, or the provision of assistive devices such as adaptive eating utensils or wheelchairs. Despite the potential for allied health professionals to assist people with HD, therapies are not always provided [31].

The gait disorders in HD include reduction in speed due to a decreased step length and cadence, an increased base of support, and an increased variability of step length, swing, and double-limb support time [12]. People with HD may have difficulty turning and with gait in dual tasks, and delays in gait initiation (akinesia) [29] resulting in a loss of independence in walking.

Training people with HD to allocate their attention effectively while carrying out tasks when walking may also be beneficial [25]. Patients have difficulty synchronizing their stepping to a cue, and there is inconsistency in the literature as to whether the cues result in short-term improvements in cadence, step, and stride length [29, 32]. The prescription of gait aids may be useful for people with HD, but the difficulty with allocating attention to a dual task and difficulty controlling the gait aid if chorea is severe could be a problem [20].

At this stage there will probably be impairment of the respiratory function and capacity, resulting in limitations in endurance and restrictions in functional activities [21].

At-home visits are important to assess the patient's functional abilities and their home environment. Recommendations for equipment or modifications are made to optimize independence and safety educating the person and her family about changes and the consequent impact on function may be useful.

Late Stages of HD

In the later stages people with HD frequently require assistance to complete basic bathing, grooming, dressing, mobility, and eating tasks [31]; the complications may include muscle contracture, pain and skin breakdowns because of the abnormal position associated with dystonia and rigidity. If there is a risk of aspiration, the physiotherapist will work closely with the speech pathologist to teach the person how to clear sputum and cough effectively [16].

Aspiration pneumonia could occur and respiratory dysfunctions may worsen. There is a decrease in exercise tolerance and the ability to perform functional activities such as ambulation. It is important to implement positioning that promotes safe swallowing, prevents secondary impairments of muscle contracture and skin breakdowns. Specialized seating, wheelchairs and hoists for transfers may need to be prescribed in the late stages of the disease [20]. Caregivers should be trained to assist with airway clearance techniques such as deep breathing, postural positioning, and supported coughing, which can be taught to the family and other staff who may be caring for the person with HD [16].

In the late stages of the disease, caregivers may find that they cannot provide the required care at home and residential care may be required. Predictors for requiring institutional care include reduced capacity to complete activities of daily living and poor motor function [33].

In conclusion, there is very little evidence evaluating the efficacy of physiotherapy, randomized control studies in the published literature for reducing impairment or increasing activity and participation in people with HD. There is evidence, however, that exercise may be useful in addressing specific impairments in people who are not severely affected by HD. A specialized multidisciplinary team is useful for identifying a program of treatment at all stages of HD.

Speech and Language Therapy in Huntington's Disease

Disorders of speech, language, and swallowing, are found in different degrees of manifestation in the course of Huntington's disease (HD). They are caused by motor, cognitive and behavioral changes, which in different combinations, can have an impact on communication and the feeding of patients. Basal ganglia degeneration, especially of the striatum, is the characteristic neuropathological finding in HD. These structures have long been known for their role in normal voluntary movement and also for causing movement disorders when damaged. However, dysfunctions in this area have also been related to different cognitive and behavioral functions, including learning, language, and social behavior [34, 35], because of its numerous connections with several cortical areas, especially the frontal lobe. Thus, in HD, extensive symptomatology is present, including motor, cognitive, and behavioral findings.

Among the motor manifestations of HD, dysarthria is a very characteristic symptom, which appears early in the course of the disease. It refers to changes in speech, caused by a disturbance in muscle control, which affects the motor bases of speech: respiration, phonation, articulation, prosody (melody and accentuation of speech), and resonance.

In HD, the changes in speech are the result of excessive involuntary movements that disturb the rate and quality of motor activities involved in speech production, featuring a hyperkinetic dysarthria pattern. According to Darley et al. [36], its main manifestation is the prosodic disorder, which may be characterized either by prosodic excess, with prolonged intervals, inappropriate pauses, and excessive accentuation of words, or prosodic insufficiency, with monopitch and monoloudness, reduced word stress, and use of short sentences. Patients with HD also have other speech characteristics, namely:

– Irregular articulation production, fast-moving and tension during phonation
– Vowel and consonant distortions

- Phonatory instability, with excessive variation of fundamental frequency
- Tense-strangled or rough voice quality
- Excessive variation in vocal intensity
- Prolonged phonemes
- Poor respiratory support for the production of speech, sometimes with apparent respiratory incoordination

In addition to speech impairments, individuals with HD have manifested changes in language comprehension and production, in its various aspects, even in the presymptomatic phase of Huntington's disease [37–40].

Some common findings in the early stages of HD are changes in spontaneous speech, with loss of conversational initiative and dysarthria [41]. At this stage, however, speech problems, in most cases, do not cause limitations in communication ability. As the disease develops, changes are described related to the reduction of the syntactic complexity of oral production [42–45], lexico-semantic deficits [46], visual naming difficulties [47, 48], and verbal comprehension deficits [43, 49, 50]. Changes in phonological and semantic verbal fluency tests are also observed [51–55]. In patients with more advanced cognitive changes, vague conversational style is observed, with reduced content.

It is important to note that language and communication difficulties are strongly linked with global cognitive impairment, which affects more clearly, in the early stages of the disease, the functions related to the frontostriatal system [41, 56]. Thus, problems are also seen in attentional and executive functions, working memory, problem-solving, visual–spatial perceptual processing, and arithmetic [37, 38, 46, 54, 57]. As the condition develops, the neuropsychological changes that affect patients fit the profile of subcortical dementia first described by Albert et al. [58], with overall slowness of intellectual activities, forgetfulness, personality changes (apathy, depression, irritability), and difficulty in manipulating acquired knowledge.

The main changes found include:

- Loss of conversational initiative and reduced spontaneous language production
- Difficulty in starting and maintainiing a topic of conversation
- Perseverence with ideas
- Reduced phrase length and message complexity
- Difficulty with lexical access
- Difficulty in maintaining face-to-face conversation, which requires integrated information processing
- Inability to pay attention to a speaker's signs and to recognize facial expressions, changes in tone of voice, and ambiguity
- Difficulty in understanding abstract, complex concepts
- Difficulty in organizing thoughts, learning and retaining new information
- Slow information processing
- Impaired auditory attention, concentration, and motivation

In HD, swallowing disruptions usually occur in the later stages of the disease, in which several aspects may be impaired (oral, pharyngeal, and esophageal phases), caused by the presence of involuntary movements that affect the muscles involved in the feeding function [59].

Dysphagia may be defined as any disruption in the eating process, from the oral cavity to the stomach [60].

In HD, swallowing disruptions usually occur in the later stages of the disease, in which several aspects may be impaired (oral, pharyngeal, and esophageal phases), caused by the presence of involuntary movements which affect the muscles involved in the feeding function [61].

In the oral phase, irregular, uncoordinated tongue movements may make it difficult to chew and control the food in the oral cavity, leading to premature spilling on the base of the tongue before a swallow reflex is triggered, increasing the risk of food aspiration. The lip seal is often ineffective and there are oral residues after swallowing.

In the pharyngeal phase, irregular movements and poor coordination of the vocal folds and the respiratory muscles, in addition to postural changes (hyperextension of the neck), may impair the airway defense mechanisms. Patients also manifest changes in pharyngeal peristalsis and esophageal motility. Multiple swallows, pharyngeal residue, coughing, choking, changes in vocal pattern, and reduced saturation during or after swallowing are also found.

Other frequent symptoms of HD are eating too fast, sudden lingual movement, respiratory chorea (involuntary respiratory movements while swallowing), eructation, aerophagia, and airway penetration of food.

Therapy for speech and language disorders is aimed at improving functional communication, in addition to intelligibility and naturalness of speech, which are aspects related to vocal intensity and/or articulation precision and to the rate of speech and/or prosodic patterns respectively [62]. Dysphagia treatment enables efficient, safe oral intake.

Current literature shows that even degenerative diseases can benefit from appropriate guidance and selections of behavioral techniques and physiological approaches in the management of patients, including relieving symptoms, especially if the intervention is multidisciplinary. Regarding HD, there are literature reviews that make broad recommendations on the best approach to speech therapy for these patients. However, we can make use of established methods, techniques, and strategies to control symptoms and maintain communication and oral intake for as long as possible.

It is important to note that to establish the best therapeutic direction, it is necessary to carry out an assessment, which will allow understanding of the symptoms, both from a motor and a functional perspective. The examination must focus on the oral sensory–motor system and neurovegetative functions—breathing chewing, and swallowing—in addition to phonation, articulation, and resonance. A detailed analysis of swallowing is of fundamental importance and for that, in addition to the evaluation of the oral sensory–motor system, patients must go through a functional assessment with food. When necessary, the clinical evaluation must be associated with additional tests, such as endoscopic evaluation of swallowing and videofluoroscopy. We found several protocols in the literature to assess dysarthria and dysphagia, some of which are specific to HD, such as the Huntington's Disease Dysphagia Scale [63]. Whenever necessary, cognitive deficits may be characterized through specific language and neuropsychological examination. The Unified Huntington's Disease Rating Scale (UHDRS), which investigates not only motor functions, but also behavioral functions, cognitive abnormalities, and functional capacity, can be used to assess the patient's cognitive status and progression over time [64].

In general, speech therapy with emphasis on the phonoarticulatory, is aimed at increasing articulatory precision, improving prosody, and reducing phonatory and respiratory instability. As the presence of chorea movements can vary, there may be periods of speech intelligibility, which tends to worsen as choreic movements increase, affecting the muscles of respiration, phonation, and articulation.

Regarding respiratory issues, pneumophonoarticulatory coordination exercises are used to improve awareness of the relationship between breathing and speaking, and also to practice inspiration and expiration control, which is related to vocal output and speech. It also seeks to train the maintenance of vocal quality and intensity, in addition to pauses (breathing and phonation), which are responsible for performance of good prosody. The oral airflow direction techniques and emissions in maximum phonation time also help to reduce the perception of hypernasality, which may occur in some cases.

When there is glottal hyperadduction, the usually tense strangled vocal quality is reduced through relaxation techniques focusing on the laryngeal muscles and using softer vocal attacks [65]. Among the therapeutic approaches that have been used, we can highlight the masticatory method [66], the yawn–sigh technique, and tongue popping with nasal sounds. The "sigh" may be used along with the production of lax vowels and words and phrases starting with vowels [62]. Chant talk techniques and exercises of voiceless fricatives followed by voiced fricatives in association with words and phrases may also be applied. Supporting sounds in ascending and descending scales and musical scales may be interesting for promoting more variations in speech frequency and intensity.

Regarding articulatory training, exercises can be performed to improve the amplitude of movement of patients' orofacial structures, especially the lips and tongue, also using over-articulation techniques. In hyperkinetic dysarthrophonia cases, plosive consonants are often uttered instead of fricatives and voiceless sounds because of the hypercontraction of the vocal folds [65]. Therefore, it may be necessary to practice points and manners of articulation of different phonemes, especially plosives and fricatives, depending on which distortions manifest in patients.

Regarding changes in speaking rate, in addition to practicing prosody, therapists may work with metronomes or hand-clapping to pace the exercises, also producing or reading words, phrases, and paragraphs stressing the tonic syllable or working with different intonations and melodies (imperative, declarative, and interrogative sentences; practicing excitement, surprise, and sadness indicators, among others).

During exercises, it is interesting that the patient can monitor his/her production through auditory and visual training, with recordings of his speech and mirror use, if he/she feels comfortable.

Speech and language therapy is also aimed at stimulating cognitive skills, especially language, through activities involving attention, concentration, reasoning, reading and writing, and interpretation. This can be accomplished through board games, computer games, paper-and-pencil activities, and reading and discussing books, in addition to constantly encouraging discursive production. Activities that require recognition, judgment, comparison, categorization, association, analysis and decision-making, logic, and problem-solving also improve thinking skills and stimulate language production. Therapists may also encourage verbal fluency and lexical access skills, which are usually impaired by executive loss. In more severe cases, the use of supplementary and alternative communication, such as printed alphabet and boards with pictures, should be encouraged.

The therapeutic approach to oropharyngeal dysphagia has the goal of stabilizing swallowing, maintaining the patients' nutritional status and pleasure of eating, in addition to preserving their lungs. To accomplish this, therapists carry out direct and indirect work.

Indirect therapy is conducted through exercises aiming to stimulate the oropharyngeal structures that take part in swallowing dynamics, improving motility, muscle tone, and sensitivity, and improving oral motor control. Direct therapy involves training with food, performing adjustments regarding consistency (such as adding thickeners to liquids), volume, speed, and other methods, including the use of adapted utensils and environmental control during feeding. Therapy also includes postural maneuvers, such as tilting the head down, and facilitating maneuvers, such as the Mendelsohn maneuver, voluntary coughing, swallowing with effort, and multiple swallows, which improve airway protection during swallowing and help to clean the pharyngeal recess.

It is important to highlight that patients with preserved cognition respond better to therapy, and therefore the treatment should start in the early stages of the disease, so that they can learn and automate appropriate behaviors and compensatory strategies for feeding and swallowing.

The choice of treatment depends on the stage and the difficulties the patient is presenting. Montagut et al. [67] suggest a rehabilitation program that includes orolingual–mandibular praxias, in addition to the training of strategies and postural changes.

Oral feeding should be maintained for as long as compensations and adaptations are possible. Once the therapist detects risks in offering food via oral intake, alternative feeding methods should be considered. In these cases, enteral nutrition is usually the preferred method. A nasogastric tube may be used in the short term, whereas for long-term treatment percutaneous endoscopic gastrostomy is the more frequently recommended method [59]. It is important to highlight that feeding care is not restricted to preventing bronchoaspiration, it is also intended to ensure that patients receive appropriate nutrition and hydration. In the case of reduced food intake, or when oral feeding is contraindicated, medical and nutritional counseling are necessary to ensure better decision-making and conduct.

It should be pointed out that training caregivers is also part of the therapeutic process, as they become increasingly responsible for establishing communication and managing or offering food to patients, once the disease starts to worsen. Their guidance is an important part of the therapeutic process, in addition to adaptation and environmental control (such as reducing distractions during communication and feeding, and using external cues to encourage swallowing).

It should also be pointed out that the type of intervention, both in dysphagia and in relation to speech and language, depends on what stage the HD patient is at and the nonlinguistic deficits associated with it— whether motor, cognitive, or psychiatric. The combination of symptoms is what makes each patient manifest unique characteristics, which influence the type of strategy that should be adopted. Additionally, because HD is a progressive disease, it is possible that at some point rehabilitation techniques will only have a limited impact. Therapists should be able to identify that point, reformulating the goals of treatment as the disease progresses and always trying to alleviate the current problems and anticipate future problems, for better adaptation of patients and their families.

References

1. Huntington's Disease Collaborative Research Group. A Novel gene containing a trinucleotide repeat that is expanded and unstable on Huntington's disease chromosomes. The Huntington's Disease Collaborative Research Group. Cell. 1993;72:971–83.
2. Craufurd D, MacLeod R, Frontali M, Quarrell O, Bijlsma EK, Davis M, et al. Diagnostic genetic testing for Huntington's disease. Pract Neurol. 2015;15:80–4.
3. Cardoso F. Huntington disease and other choreas. Neurol Clin. 2009;27:719–36.
4. Grimbergen YA, Knol MJ, Bloem BR, Kremmer BPH, Ross RAC, Munnek M. Falls and gait disturbances in Huntington's disease. Mov Disord. 2008;23:970–6.
5. Nelson AB, Kreitzer AC. Reassessing models of basal ganglia function and dysfunction. Annu Rev Neurosci. 2014;37:117–35. doi:10.1146/annurev-neuro-071013-013916.
6. Reilmann R. Pharmacological treatment of chorea in Huntington's disease—good clinical practice versus evidence-based guideline. Mov Disord. 2013;28:1030–3.
7. Armstrong MJ, Miyasaki JM. Evidence-based guideline: pharmacologic treatment of chorea in Huntington disease: report of the guideline development subcommittee of the american academy of neurology. Neurology. 2012;79:597–603.
8. Jankovic J, Roos RAC. Chorea associated with Huntington's disease: to treat or not to treat? Mov Disord. 2014;29:1414–18.
9. Wojtecki L, Groiss SJ, Ferrea S, Elben S, Hartmann CJ, Dunnett SB, Rosser A, Saft C, Südmeyer M, Ohmann C, Schnitzler A and Vesper J for the Surgical Approaches Working Group of the European Huntington's Disease Network (EHDN). A prospective pilot trial for pallidal deep brain stimulation in Huntington's disease. Front Neurol. 2015;6:177. doi:10.3389/fneur.2015.00177.
10. Gonzalez V, Cif L, Biolsi B, Garcia-Ptacek S, Seychelles A, Sanrey E, et al. Deep brain stimulation for Huntington's disease: long-term results of a prospective open-label study. J Neurosurg. 2014;121:114–22.

11. Fasano A, Mazzone P, Piano C, Quaranta D, Soleti F, Bentivoglio AR. GPi-DBS in Huntington's disease: results on motor function and cognition in a 72-year-old case. Mov Disord. 2008;23:1289–92.
12. Rao AK, Muratori L, Louis ED, Moskowitz CB, Marder KS. Spectrum of gait impairments in presymptomatic and symptomatic Huntington's disease. Mov Disord. 2008;23:1100–7.
13. Quinn L, Khalil H, Dawes H, Fritz NE, Kegelmeyer D, Kloos AD, Gillard JW, Busse M. Reliability and minimal detectable change of physical performance measures in individuals with pre-manifest and manifest Huntington disease. Phys Ther. 2013;93:942–56. doi:10.2522/ptj.20130032.
14. Jacobs JV, Boyd JT, Hogarth P, Horak F. Domains and correlates of clinical balance impairment associated with Huntington's disease. Gait Posture. 2015;41:867–70.
15. Busse ME, Wiles CM, Rosser AE. Mobility and falls in people with Huntington's disease. J Neurol Neurosurg Psychiatry. 2009;80:88–90.
16. Bilney B, Pearce A. Rehabilitation of Huntington's disease. In: Iansek R, Morris M, editors. Rehabilitation in movement disorders. Cambridge: Cambridge University Press; 2013.
17. Busse ME, Khalil H, Quinn L, Rosser AE. Physical therapy intervention for people with Huntington disease. Phys Ther. 2008;88:820–31.
18. Bilney B, Morris ME, Churchyard A, Chiu E, Georgiou-Karistianis N. Evidence for a disorder of locomotor timing in Huntington's disease. Mov Disord. 2005;20(1):51–7.
19. Goldberg A, Schepens SL, Feely SME, Garbern JY, Miller LJ, Siskind CE, Conti GE. Deficits in stepping response time are associated with impairments in balance and mobility in people with Huntington disease. J Neurol Sci. 2010;298:91–5.
20. Quinn L, Busse M. Physical therapy clinical guidelines for Huntington's disease. Neurodegener Dis Manag. 2012;2(1):21–31.
21. Kloss AD, Fritz NE, Kostyk SK, Young GS. Clinimetric properties of the Tinetti Mobility Test, Four Square Step Test, Activities-specific Balance Confidence Scale, and spatiotemporal gait measures in individuals with Huntington's disease. Gait Posture. 2014;40:647–51.
22. Bohlen S, Ekwall C, Hellstro K, Vesterlin H, Björnefur M, Wiklund L, Reilmann R. Physical therapy in Huntington's disease—toward objective assessments? Eur J Neurol. 2013;20:389–93. doi:10.1111/j.1468-1331.2012.03760.x.
23. Quinn L, Busse M, Broad M, Dawes H, Ekwall C, Fritz N, et al. European Huntington's Disease Network Physical Therapy Guidance Document. 2009. http://www.huntingtonswa.org.au/resourses/physicaltherapy-guidance-doc-2009.pdf.
24. Capato TTC. Fisioterapia. In: Qualiguato EMAB and Marques MGN editors. Doença de Huntington: Guia para familiares e profissionais da área da Saúde. 1edn. Atibaia; 2009. p. 94–105.
25. Capato TTC, Haddad MS, Piemonte MEP, Barbosa ER. Effectiveness of a physiotherapy programme, including external cues and exercises to improve gait, balance and functional independence in Huntington's disease. World Congress In Huntington's Disease. 2013;2:356. doi:10.3233/JHD-139005.
26. Capato TT d C, Tornai J, Ávila P, Barbosa ER, Piemonte MEP. Randomized controlled trial protocol: balance training with rhythmical cues to improve and maintain balance control in Parkinson's disease. BMC Neurol. 2015;15:162. doi:10.1186/s12883-015-0418-x.
27. Khalil H, Quinn L, van Deursen R, Martin R, Rosser A, Busse M. Adherence to use of a home-based exercise DVD in people with Huntington disease: participants' perspectives. Phys Ther. 2012;92(1):69–82. doi:10.2522/ptj.20100438.
28. Busse M, et al. Supporting physical activity engagement in people with Huntington's disease (ENGAGE-HD): study protocol for a randomized controlled feasibility trial. Trials. 2014;15:487. doi:10.1186/1745-6215-15-487.
29. Delval A, Krystlowiak P, Delliaux M, Dujardin K, Blatt JL, Destée A, Derambure P, Defebvre L. Role of attentional resources on gait performance in Huntington's disease. Mov Disord. 2008;23:684–9. doi:10.1002/mds.21896.
30. Hart EP, Marinus J, Burgunder JM, Bentivoglio AR, Craufurd D, Reilmann R, Saft C, Roos RAC, REGISTRY Investigators of the European Huntington's Disease Network. Better global

and cognitive functioning in choreatic versus hypokinetic-rigid Huntington's disease. Mov Disord. 2013;28(8):1142–5.

31. Bilney B, Morris ME, Perry A. Effectiveness of physiotherapy, occupational therapy, and speech pathology for people with Huntington's disease: a systematic review. Neurorehabil Neural Repair. 2003;17:12. doi:10.1177/0888439002250448.
32. Delval A, Krystlowiak P, Delliaux M, Blatt JL, Derambure P, Destée A, Defebvre L. Effect of external cueing on gait in Huntington s disease. Mov Disord. 2008;23:1446–52. doi:10.1002/mds.22125.
33. Rosenblatt A, Kumar BV, Margolis RL, Welsh CS, Ross CA. Factors contributing to institutionalization in patients with Huntington's disease. Mov Disord. 2011;26(9):1711–16. doi:10.1002/mds.23716.
34. Richfield EK, Twyman R, Berent S. Neurological syndrome following bilateral damage to the head of the caudadte nuclei. Ann Neurol. 1987;22:768–71.
35. Teichmann M, Dupoux E, Casaro P, Bachoud-Lévi AC. The role of the striatumin sentence processing: evidence from a priming study in early stages of Huntington's disease. Neuropsychologia. 2008;46(1):174–85.
36. Darley FL, Aronson AE, Brown JR. Alteraciones motrices del habla. Buenos Aires: Editorial Médica Panamericana; 1978.
37. Lemiere J, Decruyenaere M, Evers-Kiebooms G, Vandenbussche E, Dom R. Longitudinal study evaluating neuropsychological changes in so-called asymptomatic carriers of Huntington's disease mutation after 1 year. Acta Neurol Scand. 2002;106:131–41.
38. Lemiere J, Decruyenaere M, Evers-Kiebooms G, Vandenbussche RD. Cognitive changes in patients with Huntington's disease (HD) and asymptomatic carriers of the HD mutation. A longitudinal follow-up study. J Neurol. 2004;251:935–42.
39. Robins Wahlin TB, Luszcz MA, Wahlin A, Byrne GJ. Nonverbal and verbal fluency in prodromal Huntington's disease. Dement Geriatr Cogn Dis Extra. 2015;5(3):517–29.
40. Williams JK, Kim JL, Downing N, Farias S, Harrington DL, Long LD, Mills JA, Paulsen J. Everyday cognition in prodromal Huntington's disease. Neuropsychology. 2015;29(2):255–67.
41. Podoll K, Caspary P, Lange HW, Noth J. Language functions in Huntington's disease. Brain. 1988;111:1475–503.
42. Illes J. Neurolinguistic feature of spontaneous language production dissociate three forms of neurodegenerative disease: Alzheimer's, Huntington's, and Parkinson's. Brain Lang. 1989;37:628–42.
43. Murray LL. Spoken language production in Huntington's and Parkinson's disease. J Speech Lang Hear Res. 2000;43:1350–66.
44. Murray LL, Lenz LP. Productive syntax abilities in Huntington's and Parkinson's diseases. J Speech Lang Hear Res. 2001;213–19.
45. Sambin S, Teichmann M, de Diego Balaguer R, Giavazzi M, Sportiche D, Schlenker P, Bachoud-Lévi AC. The role of the striatum in sentence processing: disentangling syntax from working memory in Huntington's disease. Neuropsychologia. 2012;50(11):2625–35.
46. Smith S, Butters N, White R, Lyon L, Granholm E. Priming semantic relations in patients with Huntington's disease. Brain Lang. 1988;33:27–40.
47. Hodges JR, Salmon DP, Butters N. The nature of the naming deficit in Alzheimer's and Huntington's disease. Brain. 1991;114:1547–58.
48. Frank EM, McDade HL, Scott WK. Naming in dementia secondary to Parkinson's, Huntington's, and Alzheimer's disease. J Commun Disord. 1996;29:183–97.
49. Hanes KR, Andrews DG, Pantelis C. Cognitive flexibility and complex integration in Parkinson's disease, Huntington's disease and schizophrenia. J Int Neuropsychol Soc. 1995;1:545–53.
50. Bachoud-Lévi AC, Maison P, Bartolomeu P, Boissé MF, Barba GD, Ergis AM, Baudic S, Degos JD, Cesaro P, Peschanski M. Retest effects and cognitive decline in longitudinal follow-up of patients with early HD. Neurology. 2001;56:1052–8.

51. Bayles KA, Tomoeda CK. Confrontation naming impairment in dementia. Brain Lang. 1983;19:98–114.
52. Butters N, Wolfe J, Granholm E, Martone M. An Assessment of verbal recall, e cognition and fluency abilities in patients with Huntington's disease. Cortex. 1986;22:11–32.
53. Rosser A, Hodges JR. Initial letter and semantic category fluency in Alzheimer's disease, Huntington's disease, and progressive supranuclear palsy. J Neurol Neurosurg Psychiatry. 1994;57:1389–94.
54. Lawrence AD, Hodges JR, Rosser AE, Kershaw A, Ffrench-Constant C, Rubinsztein DC, Robbins TW, Sahakian BJ. Evidence for specific cognitive deficits in preclinical Huntington's disease. Brain. 1998;121:1329–41.
55. Azambuja MJ, Haddad MS, Radanovic M, Barbsa ER, Mansur LL. Semantic, phonologic, and verb fluency in Huntington's disease. Dement Neuropsychol. 2007;1(4):381–5.
56. Azambuja MJ, Radanovic M, Haddad MS, Adda CC, Barbosa ER, Mansur LL. Language impairment in Huntington's disease. Arq Neuropsiquiatr. 2012;70:6.
57. Lawrence AD, Watkins LHA, Sahakian BJ, Hodges JR, Robbins TW. Visual object and visuo-spatial cognition in Huntington's disease: implications for information processing in corticos-triatal circuits. Brain. 2000;123:1349–64.
58. Albert ML, Feldman RG, Willis A. The "subcortical dementia" of progressivesupranuclear palsy. J Neurol Neurosurg Psychiatry. 1974;37:121–30.
59. Zukiewicz-Sobczak W, Król R, Wróblewska P, Piatek J, Gibas-Dorna M. Huntington disease—principles and practice of nutritional management. Neurol Neurochir Pol. 2014;48(6):442–8.
60. Logemann J. Evaluation and treatment of swallowing disorders. Austin: Pro-Ed; 1983.
61. Groher ME. Dyasphagia: diagnosis and management. Newton: Butterworth-Heinemann; 1992.
62. Carrara-De Angelis E, Barros APB. Reabilitação Fonouadiológica das Disartrofonias. In: Ortiz, KZ (org). Distúrbios Neurológicos Adquiridos: fala e deglutição. Editora Manoel; 2010.
63. Heemskerk AW, Verbist B, Marinus H, Heijnen B, Sjogren E, Ross R. The Huntington's Disease Dysphagia Scale (HDDS) for measuring dysphagia in Huntington's disease patients. J Huntingtons Dis. Article first published online: 23 May 2014.
64. Toh EA, MacAskill MR, Dalrymple-Alford JC, Myall DJ, Livingston L, Macleod AS, Anderson TJ. Comparison of cognitive and UHDRS measures in monitoring disease progression in Huntington's disease: a 12-month longitudinal study. Transl Neurodegener. 2014;3:15.
65. Mourão LF. Intervenção Fonoaudiológica nos Distúrbios do Movimento. In Ortiz, KZ (org). Distúrbios Neurológicos Adquiridos: fala e deglutição. Editora Manoel; 2010.
66. Froeschels E. Chewing method as therapy. Arch Otolaryngol. 1952;56:427–34.
67. Montagut N, Gazulla D, Barreiro S, Munõz E. A disfagia em La enfermedad de Huntington: propuesta de intervención logopédica. Rev logop foniatr audiol (Ed impr) abr-jun. 2014;34(2):81–4.

Movement Disorders in Pediatrics

9

Marcelo Masruha Rodrigues and Mariana Callil Voos

Introduction

Pediatric movement disorders (MDs) is a relatively new and growing field of child neurology. Although hypokinetic disorders such as Parkinson's disease predominate in adults, children more commonly demonstrate hyperkinetic disorders, such as tics, tremor, chorea, and dystonia [1]. Furthermore, MDs in children differ from those in adults in many other aspects. Perhaps the most important is that MDs in childhood are primarily symptoms of other diseases, rather than diseases in themselves [2].

The terminology of MDs has been well defined for adults, but less so for children. Therefore, it is likely that MDs are under-reported in children, and that there is inconsistent terminology. Recently, there have been attempts to provide specific definitions of childhood motor disorders (Table 9.1) [3–5].

According to these definitions, childhood disorders can be divided into three major categories: hypertonic disorders, hyperkinetic disorders, and negative signs. Hypertonic disorders include spasticity, dystonia, and rigidity. Hyperkinetic disorders encompass chorea, dystonia, athetosis, myoclonus, tremor, stereotypies, and tics. Negative signs consist of weakness, reduced selective motor control, ataxia, apraxia, and developmental dyspraxia, although these are not discussed here [2].

In adult MDs, it is frequently helpful to divide disorders into primary and secondary disorders, although there is no consistent definition of these terms. Many authors refer to disorders as primary if there is only a single dominant symptom, and the underlying cause is presumably genetic or an identified gene. However, the

M.M. Rodrigues, M.D., Ph.D. (✉)
Division of Child Neurology, Universidade Federal de São Paulo, São Paulo, Brazil
e-mail: marcelomasruha@gmail.com

M.C. Voos, P.T., Ph.D.
Department of Physical Therapy, Faculdade de Medicina da Universidade
de São Paulo, São Paulo, Brazil
e-mail: ftmarivoos@gmail.com

© Springer International Publishing Switzerland 2017
H.F. Chien, O.G.P. Barsottini (eds.), *Movement Disorders Rehabilitation*,
DOI 10.1007/978-3-319-46062-8_9

Table 9.1 Terminology of pediatric movement disorders [3–5]

Hypertonia: abnormally increased resistance to externally imposed movement about a joint. It may be caused by spasticity, dystonia, rigidity, or a combination of features

Spasticity: a velocity-dependent resistance of a muscle to stretch. One or both of the following signs may be present:

1. Resistance to externally imposed movement increases with increasing speed of the stretch and varies with the direction of joint movement, and/or
2. Resistance to externally imposed movement rises rapidly above a threshold speed or joint angle

Dystonia: a movement disorder in which involuntarily sustained or intermittent muscle contractions cause twisting and repetitive movements, abnormal postures, or both

Rigidity: hypertonia in which all of the following are true:

1. The resistance to externally imposed joint movement is present at a very low speed, and does not exhibit a speed or angle threshold
2. Simultaneous co-contraction of agonists and antagonists may occur, and this is reflected in an immediate resistance to a reversal of the direction of movement about a joint
3. The limb does not tend to return toward a particular fixed posture or extreme joint angle
4. Voluntary activity in distant muscle groups does not lead to involuntary movements about the rigid joints, although rigidity may worsen

Chorea: an ongoing random-appearing sequence of one or more discrete involuntary movements or movement fragments

Athetosis: a slow, continuous, involuntary writhing movement that prevents maintenance of a stable posture

Myoclonus: a sequence of repeated, often nonrhythmic, brief shock-like jerks due to sudden involuntary contraction or relaxation of one or more muscles

Tremor: a rhythmic back-and-forth or oscillating involuntary movement about a joint axis

Tics: repeated, individually recognizable, intermittent movements or movement fragments that are almost briefly suppressible and are usually associated with an awareness of an urge to perform the movement

Stereotypies: repetitive, simple movements that can be voluntarily suppressed

existence of a single symptom in childhood MDs is probably the exception rather than the rule [2].

As this is a book that deals with rehabilitation of MDs, we discuss the disorders that are of interest in pediatrics: cerebral palsy and dystonia.

Cerebral Palsy

The term "cerebral palsy" constitutes a useful socio-medical framework for certain motor disabled children with special needs. However, it does not describe a single disease entity but rather a collection of disorders with different etiologies [6].

Cerebral palsy (CP) is defined as "a group of disorders of the development of movement and posture, causing activity limitation, that are attributed to non-progressive disturbances that occurred in the developing fetal or infant brain" [7]. Virtually all such disturbances occur during or before early infancy. Although tone and postural abnormalities may become more pronounced during early childhood, qualitative evolution is uncommon. The full extent of motor disability may not be evident until the age of 3 or 4 years [8]. Intellectual, sensory, and behavioral difficulties may accompany CP, and are especially common in patients with spastic quadriplegia and severe motor disability [9].

Children with CP often exhibit mental retardation (52 %), hearing impairment (12 %), and speech and language disorders (38 %) [10], in addition to congenital anomalies [11]. Epilepsy occurs in 34–94 % of children with CP, depending on the study population. Although neurological impairment beyond the motor involvement frequently occurs, the diagnosis of CP rests upon the presence of motor disability alone [8].

Cerebral palsy occurs in 1.2–3.6 children per 1,000 live births [8]. Numerous CP registries exist throughout the world, and population prevalence rates from four continents have remained consistent over several decades [12]. Prematurity is the single most important risk factor for CP. The risk of CP in very low birth weight infants is as high as 4–10 %, whereas the risk in term infants is only 1–0,1% live births [13].

Attempts at classification of CP have been multiple and no system has been completely satisfactory. An etiological classification is not useful because similar etiological factors can produce different topology and extent of lesions and thus different clinical features. The use of neuroimaging, and its role in the understanding of CP pathogenesis, has dramatically increased over the last 20 years. It plays an increasing role in the diagnosis of CP, and a classification according to imaging results could be considered. However, neuroimaging, and especially magnetic resonance imaging (MRI), is not consistently available in all countries; thus, comparison among countries and across time periods would be difficult, especially as normal MRI does not rule out the diagnosis of CP [6].

A clinical, phenomenological classification, therefore, is more useful than etiological or pathological ones. From a clinical viewpoint, CP is usually classified into neurologically defined subtypes: spastic, dyskinetic, and ataxic. The spastic types can in turn be subdivided according to the topography of involvement into spastic hemiplegia, spastic diplegia, and spastic quadriplegia [6].

Spastic forms of CP account for the majority (85–90 %) of cases, around one third being unilateral and two thirds bilateral; dyskinetic forms occur in around 7 % and ataxic forms in around 4 % of cases [14].

Spastic Cerebral Palsy

Spastic CP is divided into unilateral forms (hemiplegia, hemiparesis) and bilateral spastic CP. Bilateral forms in turn are divided into "leg-dominated" forms, also termed diplegia or diparesis, in which involvement of the lower limbs is dominant, and "arm-dominated" forms or quadriplegia/tetraplegia or paresis, where the upper limbs are predominantly affected or all four limbs are approximately equally involved. These forms are further subdivided into mild, moderate, and severe types, taking into account the functional severity [6].

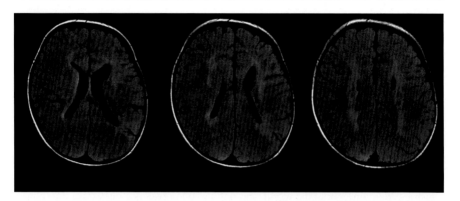

Fig. 9.1 *Periventricular leukomalacia* in a child with spastic diplegia. Axial fluid attenuation inversion recovery (FLAIR) images showing ventriculomegaly with irregular margins of bodies and trigones of the lateral ventricles, loss of periventricular white matter with increased signal, and thinning of the corpus callosum

Spastic Diplegia

The most common type of bilateral spastic CP is spastic diplegia, defined as a type in which the lower limbs are much more severely affected than the arms. Involvement of the upper limbs is constant, however, even though it may be very mild and detectable only by careful examination. Preterm infants are particularly prone to spastic diplegia. Approximately 80 % of preterm infants who manifest motor abnormalities have spastic diplegia [15]. In recent years, the survival of very small preterm infants has resulted in a larger group of more severely neurologically impaired survivors [16].

The pathology of diplegia is related to periventricular lesions, which are the predominant type of brain damage in preterm babies. Intraventricular hemorrhage, especially when followed by ventricular dilatation, is a possible cause of diplegia. Periventricular leukomalacia is the most common lesion responsible for spastic diplegia [6]. This is easily understandable, as the involved areas are located along the external angle of the lateral ventricles, thus damaging the fibers from the internal aspect of the hemisphere, which includes the motor fibers to the lower limbs (Fig. 9.1). The location of leukomalacia along the posterior part of the lateral ventricles, interrupting the optic radiations, is responsible for visual impairment [17].

Some infants with spastic diplegia manifest ataxia after further maturation. These infants have a great increase in tone of the leg muscles and accompanying difficulties in coordination and strength. Impairment may be asymmetric. When a small child is held in the vertical position by the examiner and the plantar surfaces of the feet are bounced lightly on the examining table, adduction of the legs (scissoring) and obligatory extension (extensor thrust) are seen. The feet are also kept in an equinovarus posture. Further examination reveals weakness of dorsiflexion of the feet. In older children, this same spasticity causes them to toe-walk. As expected, signs of upper motor unit involvement are easily demonstrable in the legs (e.g., hyperactive deep tendon reflexes, bilateral ankle clonus, extensor toe signs). Striking spasticity of the hip muscles may lead to subluxation of the femur and associated

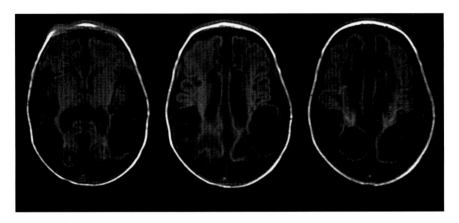

Fig. 9.2 *Multicystic encephalomalacia* in a child with spastic quadriplegia. Axial T1-weighted images showing numerous loculated, lacy pseudocysts within the white matter and cortex

acetabular pathological conditions and further restriction of motion [8]. After a variable period, usually 18 months to 2 years in children with moderate involvement, spasticity is increasingly accompanied by contractures that maintain the hips and knees in flexion, and the feet in an equinovarus position.

Spastic Quadriplegia

Spastic quadriplegia is the most severe type of CP. The condition is characterized by bilateral spasticity predominating in the upper limbs with involvement of the bulbar muscles, almost always in association with severe mental retardation and microcephaly. Quadriplegia, also termed tetraplegia, bilateral hemiplegia or four-limbed dominated CP, is less common than diplegia. Although it accounts for only 5 % of all cases of CP, it represents a significant problem, as affected children are totally dependent and pose the most difficult problems with regard to care, feeding, and prevention of deformities [6].

There is a high incidence of brain malformations in this group, and destructive processes of pre- or perinatal origin such as multicystic encephalomalacia or CNS infections are common (Fig. 9.2). The predominance of term children is confirmed in many series [14, 18, 19].

Opisthotonic posturing may be evident in early infancy and may persist throughout the first year of life. Movement of the head often initiates forced extension of the arms and legs, resulting in a position similar to that in decerebrate rigidity. Accompanying supranuclear bulbar palsy, the result of bilateral corticobulbar tract impairment, may produce difficulties with swallowing and articulation. The incoordination of the oropharyngeal muscles may predispose the patient to recurrent pneumonia during the first years of life [8].

Neurological examination demonstrates marked spasticity and accompanying signs of corticospinal tract involvement, including hyperactive deep tendon reflexes, ankle clonus, and extensor toe signs. Weakness of dorsiflexion of the feet,

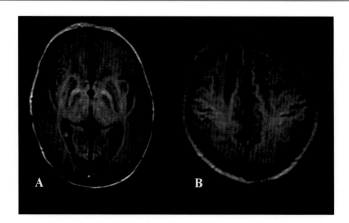

Fig. 9.3 *Selective gray matter lesions* in a child with mixed cerebral palsy (CP). Axial FLAIR images showing (**a**) basal ganglia and (**b**) perirolandic lesions. This child suffered a severe perinatal hypoxic–ischemic injury

associated with equinovarus deformities, is common. Marked spasticity of the hip muscles may lead to subluxation of the femur and associated acetabular pathological conditions. Flexion contractures of the wrists and elbows of various degrees and spasticity of the arm muscles are readily apparent [8].

The severe forms often have some dystonic features that affect the hands, face, and even trunk, so that differentiation from dystonic CP is not always clear-cut. The borderline between tetraplegia and dystonic CP may be difficult to draw, and the term spastic–dyskinetic CP reflects the possible interaction of dystonic and spastic features (Fig. 9.3).

The incidence of auditory, visual, motor, and learning disability is much higher in children with spastic quadriplegia than in children with spastic hemiplegia, spastic diplegia, or ataxic CP [9].

Spastic Hemiplegia

Although children may manifest obvious hemiplegia in the second year of life, specific difficulties may not be observed during the first 3–5 months of life. After a perinatal stroke, an infant may be neurologically normal until the development of pathological handedness at approximately 4–6 months of age. For unexplained reasons, the left hemisphere (right side of the body) is affected in two-thirds of patients, and perinatal stroke is more common on the left than on the right [20].

Spastic hemiplegia is the most common form of CP found in term-born children; around one quarter to one third of patients are born preterm [21]. The prevalence of unilateral spastic CP, or hemiplegia/hemiparesis, is reported in the European survey to be about 0.6 per 1,000 live births [14].

Neonatal stroke, which encompasses ischemic perinatal infarction and sinovenous thrombosis occurring in the perinatal period (before the age of 7 days) or the neonatal period (before 28 days of age), is a particularly important cause of CP [20]. Ischemic perinatal stroke may be responsible for 28–50 % of all cases of hemiplegic CP in term infants [22]. Obvious prenatal factors (e.g., brain malformations) were

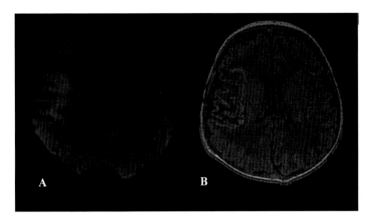

Fig. 9.4 *Perinatal ischemic stroke* in a child with hemiplegic CP. (**a**) Diffusion-weighted image and (**b**) axial T1-weighted image showing hyperintensity in the middle cerebral artery territory (*M2*)

present in 7.6 % of a cohort in one series [23], but the proportion is higher in others [24]. Obvious perinatal factors, mainly intracerebral hemorrhage, were found in 4.5 % of term and 8.1 % of preterm infants, and postnatal factors in 10.7 % of cases (Fig. 9.4). Etiology remained unspecified in one third to one quarter of cases, even though abnormal prenatal events were much more frequent in patients than in control infants [6].

During the examination, the child exhibits impaired gross and fine motor coordination, has difficulty moving the hand quickly, and is frequently unable to grasp small items with a pincer grasp. The obligate (palmar) grasp reflex, which is usually absent by the age of 6 months and frequently rudimentary after the age of 4 months, may remain obligate. Weakness of the wrist and forearm is often associated with a limited range of motion of supination. The range of elbow extension may be restricted. Attempts at reaching for objects may be accompanied by athetotic posturing with flexion of the wrist and hyperextension of the fingers (avoidance reaction). Facial involvement is unusual [8].

Only 10 % of affected patients, including those with extensive hemiplegia, have homonymous hemianopia [25]. Children with hemiparesis may have a circumduction gait with a variable degree of abnormality. Most commonly, the child walks on the toes and swings the affected leg over a nearly semicircular arc during the course of each step. In contrast with the leg, the affected arm usually moves less than normal and does not participate in normal reciprocal motion during ambulation. An equinovarus positioning of the foot is seen; weakness and a lack of full range of motion of dorsiflexion are often present. Further evidence of upper motor neuron involvement on the hemiplegic side includes hyperreflexia of the deep tendon reflexes, ankle clonus, and extensor toe signs [8].

Although frequently overlooked, corticosensory impairment and hemineglect of the affected side are common. Examination for the integrity of stereognosis and graphesthesia usually reveals varying degrees of compromise [26].

Dyskinetic Cerebral Palsy

The prevalence of dyskinetic CP (dystonic and athetoid subtypes combined) is about 0.15 per 1,000 live births [14]. It is particularly reported in term-born children [21].

Dyskinetic CP is characterized by involuntary, uncontrolled, recurring, occasionally stereotyped movements, with persistence of predominant primitive reflex patterns and varying muscle [14]. The essential disability in dystonic–dyskinetic CP is an inability to organize and properly execute intended movements, to coordinate automatic movements and to maintain a posture. This results in major disability, all the more so as primitive motor patterns, such as the asymmetrical tonic neck reflex, are usually persistent and there is often some degree of associated spasticity [6].

In the dystonic subgroup, the motor disorder is characterized by sudden, abnormal shifts of general muscle tone, especially increases in muscle tone in trunk extensors induced by emotional stimuli and changes in the posture of neck muscles in intended acts or movements. These patients also have a tendency to repeatedly assume and retain distorted, twisted postures in the same stereotypical pattern [27]. As discussed above, severe bilateral spastic CP is very often characterized by additional dyskinetic—more specifically dystonic—features.

Choreoathetotic CP is characterized by large-amplitude, involuntary movements. Athetosis usually involves the distal limbs and results in slow, writhing, involuntary movements. Chorea may involve the face, limbs, and rarely the trunk. The combination of athetoid and choreiform movements results in a pattern of distal extremity movement, on-going hypertonia, and rotary writhing movements of the limbs. Tremor, myoclonus, and even some element of dystonia may also be evident. Pure dyskinetic MDs do not feature hyperreflexia with clonus or pyramidal signs, whereas in dyskinetic CP these spastic signs may be present [8].

Dyskinetic forms of CP constitute a rather well-defined group from the etiological point of view [27]. The incidence of perinatal factors is higher than in other types of CP, with 67 % of factors referable to the perinatal period, 21 % to the prenatal period, and a small proportion of postnatally acquired or untraceable cases. Hyperkinetic cases are seen both in term infants of normal birth weight who suffer severe asphyxia at birth and in small for gestational age infants with hypoxia [28]. Among hyperkinetic cases there is a very high proportion of preterm, appropriate for gestational age, infants, some with hyperbilirubinemia, often in combination with hypoxia (Fig. 9.5).

Ataxic Cerebral Palsy

Ataxic CP, called by some authors "nonprogressive congenital ataxia" [29], occurred in 0.09 per 1,000 live births in a European series [14]. Nonprogressive ataxia is an obviously heterogeneous condition. Its pathogenic mechanisms are poorly known and its nosological interpretation is controversial. The term is used here to designate only those cases in which cerebellar symptoms and signs are clearly at the forefront.

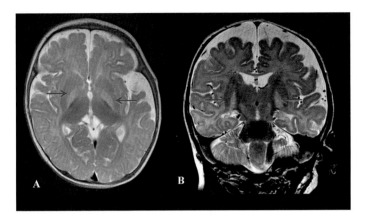

Fig. 9.5 *Kernicterus* in a child with dyskinetic CP. (**a**) Axial T2-weighted image shows bilateral pallidal hyperintensity (*arrows*) and (**b**) coronal T2-weighted image shows bilateral pallidal and subthalamic hyperintensity (*arrowheads*)

Most cases of nonprogressive cerebellar ataxia are congenital, even though the clinical manifestations often do not become suggestive before 1 or 2 years of age, at the time when children normally begin to walk [6]. Prenatal factors play a dominant role in the etiology of nonprogressive cerebellar ataxia and genetic abnormalities are probably the main cause of this type of CP. Ataxia is discussed in Chap. 5.

Mixed Cerebral Palsy

Children with a combination of spastic and dyskinetic types are labeled as having a mixed type.

Management

The management of CP requires a comprehensive multidisciplinary team approach that can deal with the numerous psychological, behavioral, and physical needs of the child and family.

The goal of physical therapy is to help individuals develop coordination [30–32], build strength [33–37], improve balance [38–40], maintain flexibility [41–44], optimize physical functioning levels, and maximize independence [30, 32, 35–39, 45, 46]. Physical therapists instruct patients and families on the proper use of walkers and/or other gait adaptive equipment.

Physical therapy involves the practice of postural transferring, such as rolling, sitting, crawling, kneeling, standing and walking [36–39, 43–47]. The largest benefit of therapy to the child with CP is in the treatment of problematic conditions when they occur, including muscle atrophy or tightening [33–36], loss in joint range of motion [41–44], muscle spasticity [43, 44, 48], pain in muscles and joints, joint inflammation, and/or contractures (muscle rigidity) [43, 44].

Occupational therapists teach techniques for easier dressing and other forms of self-care. They instruct on how to use splints for the hand and/or wrist to aid in eating, or other devices to help the child to reach and/or grasp objects. The goal of therapy is to ensure that a child achieves the highest level of functional performance within their home, school, public, and work environments [30, 32].

Occupational therapy employs adaptive processes to teach a child to perform tasks required in the normal course of a day. This is accomplished by focusing on identifying adaptive methods a child can learn to complete tasks, breaking down essential tasks into smaller steps, often modified, capitalizing on the need for accomplishment, pride, enjoyment, and independence, developing in a child a sense of place in their environment, at school, and in the community [30, 32, 49, 50].

Speech therapy can be helpful in improving oral motor control and swallowing. Some children with cerebral palsy have difficulty controlling the muscles in their face, throat, neck, and head. This can lead to troubles with speech, chewing, and swallowing [51]. It can also cause drooling and affect the overall ability to interact and learn. Those who also have difficulty hearing may have a hard time understanding spoken language.

Speech and language therapy seek to improve a child's speech and communication by strengthening the muscles used for speech, increasing oral motor skills, and by improving their understanding of speech and language [51, 52]. It can also can help with swallowing disorders, such as dysphagia. Speech therapy is also helpful in addressing verbal fluency, which may be affected by both motor (oral motor control) and cognitive (memory and perception) losses [52].

Movement disorders cause not only pain and discomfort, but also depression, social isolation and low quality of life, owing to the embarrassment caused by the involuntary movements. Motor rehabilitation can minimize pain and isolation; thus, adherence to motor rehabilitation is important for achieving positive results [30, 53]. To ensure repetition and, therefore, motor learning, patients and caregivers must be instructed to practice at home the exercises performed at therapy sessions [30, 53].

Treatment should begin as early as possible, with the goal of therapy formulated to improve care, optimize motor function, prevent orthopedic deformities, and address associated impairments. Rehabilitative programs have a direct benefit for parent–child relationships, social and emotional status, confidence, and self-esteem [54].

Clinical Scales

Gross Motor Function Measure

Motor function may be assessed with Gross Motor Function Measure (GMFM). The GMFM is a widely used, criterion-referenced, clinical observation tool, with a scale from 0 to 100, that was developed and validated for children with CP. It has excellent reliability and demonstrates the ability to evaluate meaningful change in gross motor function in children diagnosed with CP [55].

The GMFM measures gross motor function when carrying out lying and roll-ing, crawling and kneeling, sitting, standing, and walk–run–jump activities. It focuses on the extent of the achievement of a variety of gross motor activities (mainly mobility skills and activities requiring postural control such as sitting, kneeling, and standing on one foot) that a typically developing 5-year-old can accomplish [55].

Gross Motor Function Classification System

Children with CP can be categorized using the Gross Motor Function Classification System (GMFCS) into five levels where level I is the greatest mobility; "the child walks without restriction: limitations in more advanced gross motor skills" to level V; "self-mobility is severely limited, even with the use of assistive technology" [56]. The GMFCS is a reliable and valid system that classifies children with CP according to their age-specific gross motor activity.

The GMFCS describes the major functional characteristics of children with CP at each level within the following age windows: before the second birthday; between the age of 2 years and the 4th birthday; between the age of 4 years and the 6th birth-day; and between the ages of 6 and 12 years.

Pediatric Evaluation of Disability Inventory

The Pediatric Evaluation of Disability Inventory (PEDI) was developed as a com-prehensive functional assessment instrument for rehabilitation. It has three domains: self-care, mobility, and social function. Caregiver assistance in complex activities and environmental modifications/equipment can be described. PEDI can be used as a parent report/structured interview instrument or by professionals observing the child's functional behavior in a hospital or outpatient setting.

The self-care domain has 73 items, mobility has 59, and social function has 65 items. There are eight questions on self-care and five on social function, scoring 5 for independent, 4 for supervised, 3 for minimal assistance, 20 for moderate assis-tance, 1 for maximum assistance, and 0 for full assistance. Lower scores mean greater dependence [57].

Spastic Cerebral Palsy Treatment

Spasticity causes muscle stiffness and weakness, and decreases daily functional activities, including standing and walking [48]. A variety of antispasticity interven-tions are available for the treatment of children with CP, including physical therapy, oral medications, neurolytic blocking agents, intrathecal baclofen pumps, tendon-lengthening procedures, and selective dorsal rhizotomy.

Physical Therapy

In general, physical therapy programs are tailored to the needs of children. Physical therapy assessment of children with CP includes history, functional level, neuromo-tor characteristics (spasticity, muscular synergies, voluntary movement description, transferring description, joint range of motion, strength), sensory systems (visual, vestibular, proprioceptive, hearing, tactile), perception, respiratory, and cardiac functions. Based on this evaluation, objectives are established and a treatment is proposed [58].

Specific treatment programs at the different levels of functional independence at a particular moment show better results than general therapy programs, but both approaches have positive effects on gait speed and gross motor function [38]. Most studies address the outcomes after physiotherapy programs for children with hemiplegia or diplegia [30, 32, 36, 37, 43, 44], but some studies also show improvement in children with quadriplegia [35, 53].

Passive Muscle Stretching

Passive muscle stretching is used for individuals with spastic CP to reduce the tightness or contracture of soft tissues. Manual stretching can increase the range of movements, reduce spasticity, and even improve walking efficiency in children with spasticity. Sustained stretching of longer duration showed greater improvement in the range of movements and reduced spasticity of muscles around targeted joints [41].

Prolonged passive muscle stretching while standing on a tilt-table decreases the resistance to passive ankle joint movements in children with CP [42]. A daily standing program with hip abduction provided acetabular development and maintained hip abduction range of motion in the spastic adductor muscles in ambulatory children with spastic diplegia CP, when performed during the first years of life [43, 44].

Muscle Strengthening by Functional Training

According to neurodevelopmental treatment principles, the motor problems of CP arise fundamentally from central nervous system dysfunction, which interferes with the development of normal postural control against gravity and impedes normal motor development [45, 59]. The goal is the establishment of normal motor development and function and/or the prevention of contractures and deformities. The approach focuses on sensorimotor components of muscle tone, reflexes and abnormal movement patterns, postural control, sensation, perception, and memory [59].

Handling techniques that control various sensory stimuli have been used to inhibit spasticity, abnormal reflexes, and abnormal movement patterns. Neurodevelopmental treatment is used to facilitate normal muscle tone, equilibrium responses, and movement patterns. The normal developmental sequence is advocated as a framework for treatment. Neurodevelopmental treatment focusing on sit-to-stand transfer enables children with spastic diplegia to perform these movements more efficiently, with selective muscle control. Results can be observed after the first session of treatment [45].

A dynamic postural stability training program improves balance control and gait parameters in children with CP. The program has eight levels of difficulty and consists in keeping balance while standing on a platform. It has resulted in improvements in stability indices and gait parameters in children with spastic CP [39].

One study showed that trunk–hip strengthening exercises are effective for improvement in trunk and hip muscle activation. The exercises also improved the position of the pelvis, with a decrease in anterior pelvic tilt motion during standing in children with spastic diplegia [37]. The association of neurodevelopmental treatment and progressive functional training can increase the muscle thickness of the quadriceps femoris and rectus femoris and improve the mobility of children with spastic CP [36].

Children with moderate to severe cerebral palsy also benefit from muscle strengthening. Children classified as IV or V in the GMFCS are at risk for low bone mass for chronological age, which compounds the risk in adulthood for progressive deformity and chronic pain. A regular program of seated speed, resistance, and power training exercises improve bone mineral density and prevent spinal deformity and back pain in adulthood [35, 56]. Some patients also report improved bowel and bladder control, and increased energy levels [35].

A daily physiotherapy program, based on motor learning principles, was feasible and improved overall development, even in children with cerebral palsy at GMFCS level V, which is the lowest motor function level [53]. After 4 consecutive weeks of 2 h of PT intervention based on motor learning principles 5 days a week, children showed improvements in motor function, language, and cognitive skills [53].

Electrical Stimulation

Electrical stimulation has been applied in children with CP to increase strength and range of motion, reduce spasticity, and improve the performance of activities [33]. Neuromuscular electrical stimulation activates muscles in isolation when aimed at reducing impairments such as weakness or spasticity, whereas threshold electrical stimulation affects muscles at subcontraction levels (often during sleep) when aimed at increasing circulation [34].

In contrast, functional electrical stimulation causes muscles to contract during the performance of an activity such as sitting, standing up from a chair, walking, or reaching for and manipulating objects [33]. Therefore, electrical stimulation has been recommended as an additional tool during functional practice of children with CP [34].

Constraint-Induced Movement Therapy and Bimanual Intense Therapy

Constraint-induced movement therapy attempts to promote hand function by using intensive practice using the affected hand while restraining the less-affected hand [32]. Impaired hand function is among the most functionally disabling symptoms of children with unilateral cerebral palsy. Recent approaches providing intensive upper extremity training are promising: constraint-induced movement therapy, when children perform tasks with the affected hand, and bimanual training (hand–arm bimanual intensive therapy), when children perform tasks that require both hands.

Constraint-induced movement therapy and bimanual training improve dexterity and bimanual upper extremity use; however, training must have a high intensity. Ninety hours of constraint-induced movement therapy and bimanual training lead to greater improvements than 60 h of the same treatments [30]. Bimanual training may allow direct practice of functionally meaningful goals, and such practice may transfer to unpracticed goals and improve bimanual coordination. Increased dosing frequency may be needed for older children and combined approaches may be useful, but require sufficient intensity.

The constraint-induced movement therapy has been recently proposed in the context of a day camp model for children aged 5–9 years with spastic hemiplegic cerebral palsy. The intervention resulted in significant improvement in distal control of the affected limb. It is interesting to mention that increased social function was also observed after the intervention. All improvements were maintained at the 3-month follow-up assessment [32].

Another recent study showed the positive effects of a home-based, intensive bimanual intervention with children with unilateral spastic cerebral palsy. Trained caregivers provided 90 h of intensive, bimanual hand–arm therapy in the home after which children demonstrated significant improvements in hand function [30].

Virtual Reality Training

Virtual reality treadmill training has been beneficial for children with spastic cerebral palsy. A study showed that gait performance improved after 8 weeks' training [46]. Treadmill gait training with virtual reality was also very effective for improving the balance abilities and muscular strength of the lower limbs and gross motor function [46].

Virtual reality training improved hand–eye coordination and visual motor speed in children with spastic cerebral palsy [31]. Motion interactive games can be a complementary tool in home rehabilitation. There was significant improvement in the motor performance of children who had home practice with the Nintendo Wii [49].

Hippotherapy

Horseback riding has been considered one of the best interventions for promoting the sitting ability of children with spastic cerebral palsy [47, 60, 61]. Park et al. [61] demonstrated the beneficial effects of hippotherapy on gross motor function and functional performance in children with CP. Previous studies have indicated the therapeutic effects of horseback riding, including improvement in postural stability, increase in sensory inputs, decrease in muscle tone, increase in range of motion, facilitation of muscle synergy, and improvement in postural muscle activities [40, 47, 60].

Aquatic Therapy

Lai et al. [62] investigated the effects of aquatic therapy on motor function, enjoyment, activities of daily living, and health-related quality of life for children with spastic CP of various motor severities. Aquatic therapy improved the scores on a 66-item GMFM, even for children with GMFCS level IV. Children treated with aquatic therapy had higher Physical Activity Enjoyment Scale scores.

Sensory Integration

Sensory integration is the main approach for children with learning difficulties, attention deficits, and autism. It focuses on the sensory aspects and has a positive impact on motivation, attention, quality of movement, and social and emotional well-being. Sensory integration principles include giving the opportunity to experience sensory stimuli, encouraging adaptive responses with sensory–motor–cognitive interaction, motivating the child to explore the environment [58].

Orthoses

Ankle–foot orthoses control equinus feet and knee hyperextension, caused by triceps spasticity. They can improve gait quality and reduce energetic demands during walking [58]. Children with spastic diplegic CP, who ambulate with excessive ankle plantar flexion during stance show improvement with bilateral ankle–foot orthoses [63].

Prescription of ankle–foot orthoses is common for patients with CP. Typical treatment objectives are to improve ankle–foot function and enhance general gait quality. Ries et al.[64] investigated the effectiveness of ankle–foot orthosis for improving the gait of children with diplegic CP. They concluded that step length exhibited clinically meaningful improvement. Orthosis design was shown to effect changes in speed and ankle function and should be investigated in future studies.

Oral Therapy

Oral therapy is usually of greater relevance for individuals with diplegic or quadriplegic CP. Several agents have been used with some benefit, including benzodiazepines, dantrolene, baclofen, and alpha-2-adrenergic-agonists (tizanidine). In general, these approaches help to reduce spasticity, but have little beneficial effect on signs of weakness and incoordination [65].

Neuromuscular Blocking Agents

Neuromuscular blocking agents, including alcohol, aqueous phenol, local anesthetics, and botulinum A toxin, have been use to improve the balance between overly spastic agonist muscles and weakened antagonist muscles. Botulinum A toxin, the most widely used agent in this category, acts by blocking acetylcholine release at the neuromuscular junction. Typically, the peak effect occurs at 2–4 weeks and reinjection is necessary at 12–14 weeks [66]. A subcommittee of the American Academy of Neurology has recommended that botulinum neurotoxin be offered as a treatment option in children and adults with spasticity [67].

Continuous intrathecal baclofen infusion through indwelling catheters and a programmable pump has been shown to reduce spasticity in the upper and lower extremities and improve function and activities of daily living [68]. Complications include infections, problems with the catheter (kinking, migration), headaches, nausea, and unresponsiveness or profound hypotonia caused by overdosing.

Intrathecal baclofen has been shown to be beneficial in dystonic CP, but not in other dyskinetic forms [69]. Typical candidates for this therapy include children with moderate to severe spastic quadriplegia in whom oral therapy has failed, those who respond to a screening bolus of medication, and those who have adequate body size for placement of the subcutaneous pump [66].

Orthopedic Surgery

The role of the orthopedic surgeon is to maintain or enhance motor abilities and to prevent deformities through procedures such as tendonotomies, muscle transfers, osteotomies, and arthrodesis. Aggressive use of botulinum A toxin, physical therapy, casting, and orthotics has effectively delayed the timing of surgical intervention to later in childhood. There is also an increasing trend toward single-event, multi-level surgery rather than sequential, more piecemeal, approaches [70].

Dyskinetic Cerebral Palsy

The treatment of dyskinetic CP is complicated, because most individuals have mixed degrees of chorea, athetosis, and dystonia. The general approach to therapy in the child with CP is to target the dyskinetic movement that is causing the greatest difficulty. Therapeutic trials are largely empirical, and responses are often individualized [65].

When the symptom is primarily chorea or athetosis, benzodiazepines, valproate, carbamazepine, tetrabenazine, and neuroleptics are often prescribed. In contrast, therapy for dystonic CP includes trials with anticholinergic medications (biperiden, trihexyphenidyl) [71], baclofen, anticonvulsants (carbamazepine, clonazepam), antiparkinsonian medications (levodopa/carbidopa), and botulinum toxin [66].

Preliminary studies have suggested that deep brain stimulation may be effective in selected patients with dystonia, and possibly choreoathetosis [72].

Dystonia

Childhood dystonia is defined as "a movement disorder in which involuntary sustained or intermittent muscle contractions cause twisting and repetitive movements, abnormal postures, or both" [4]. Dystonia can occur as an associated feature in may static and degenerative childhood disorders. Although the term seems to imply an abnormality of tone, dystonia is not primarily a disorder of tone, but rather a disorder of posture and/or movement. When individuals with dystonia are at rest, tone is often diminished, although, in severe dystonia, involuntary contractions persist during attempted rest and tone may be increased. Dystonia can manifest as hypertonic dystonia with increased stiffness, hyperkinetic dystonia with increased movement, or a combination of the two.

Dystonia can also be reflected in very slow twisting or writhing movements or very quick ballistic movements, and can have rhythmicity, appearing to be a tremor, in which case it would be referred to as dystonic tremor [2]. Causes of dystonia and dystonia-like movements in childhood are summarized in Table 9.2.

Table 9.2 Main causes of dystonia in childhood [2]

Static injury/structural disorders	*Hereditary/degenerative disorders*
Cerebral palsy	DYT1
Hypoxic–ischemic injury	DYT2
Kernicterus	DYT3
Head trauma	DYT4
Encephalitis	DYT5
Tumors	DYT6
Stroke in the basal ganglia (which may be due to vascular abnormalities or varicella)	DYT7
Congenital malformations	DYT8
Drugs/toxins	DYT9
Neuroleptic and antiemetic medications	DYT10
Calcium channel blockers	DYT11
Stimulants (amphetamine, cocaine, ergot alkaloids)	Fahr's disease
Anticonvulsants (carbamazepine, phenytoin)	Pantothenate kinase-associated neurodegeneration
Thallium	Huntington's disease
Manganese	Spinocerebellar ataxias
Carbon monoxide	Neuronal ceroid lipofuscinosis
Ethylene glycol	Rett's syndrome
Cyanide	Striatal necrosis
Methanol	Leigh's disease and other mitochondrial disorders
Wasp sting	Neuro-acanthocytosis
Paroxysmal disorders	Ataxia–telangiectasia
Paroxysmal nonkinesigenic choreoathetosis (DYT9)	Tay–Sachs disease
Paroxysmal kinesigenic choreoathetosis (DYT10)	Niemann–Pick type C
Exercise-induced dystonia	GM1 gangliosidosis
Alternating hemiplegia of childhood	Metachromatic leukodystrophy
Paroxysmal torticollis of infancy	Lesch–Nyhan disease
	Glutaric aciduria types 1 and 2
	Acyl-CoA dehydrogenase deficiencies
	Wilson's disease
	Methylmalonic aciduria

Dystonia is classified by etiology as either primary or secondary, and by distribution as focal, segmental, hemidystonia, multifocal, or generalized dystonia (Table 9.3).

Clinical Evaluation

Discriminating dystonia in children is complex and requires observation and knowledge of the disorders that may be concurrent with dystonia, such as spasticity, retractions, weakness, and bradykinesia. A neurological examination associated with clinical scales may describe and provide scores to quantify dystonia.

Table 9.3 Dystonia classification

Etiology
Primary: when it is the predominant or only clinical feature
Secondary: when it exists as just one neurological sign or symptom among others
Distribution
Focal: involves a single part of the body, such as a limb, the neck, or the face
Segmental: involves the muscles of two contiguous body parts
Hemidystonia: involves all or most muscles on one side of the body
Multifocal: involves two or more noncontiguous body regions
Generalized: involves multiple limbs on both sides of the body, including at least one leg

The Hypertonia Assessment Tool for children was developed to differentiate between the clinical features of childhood hypertonia: dystonia, spasticity, and rigidity. It consists of seven items to assess the presence/absence of hypertonic components. It is useful for both clinical and research purposes [73].

The Burke–Fahn–Marsden Movement Scale was designed with two components: a movement scale and a disability scale. It is mainly based on function and was designed to evaluate primary dystonia. The scale assesses nine body regions with regard to the severity factor and the provoking factor. The disability scale is based on the individual's assessment of how the dystonia affects activities of daily living [74].

The Barry–Albright Dystonia Scale was developed to assess children and adults who are unable to cooperate with the examination, particularly children with secondary dystonia. Patients with secondary dystonia may have cognitive deficits, may be unable to follow instructions, and often have difficulty with daily motor activities. It is a five-point ordinal scale for eight body regions: eyes, mouth, neck, trunk, left and right upper extremities, and left and right lower extremities [75].

The Unified Dystonia Rating Scale evaluates the severity and duration of excess movements in dystonia in 14 different body regions. It quantifies involuntary excess movement and does not reflect hypertonia or fixed postures. The Global Dystonia Rating Scale is a more detailed version, with a larger ordinal scale ranging from 0 to 10 instead of from 0 to 4 points for the 14 body regions [76].

Treatments for Dystonia

Oral Medication

Because dopa-responsive dystonia can mimic CP, it has been recommended that all children with unexplained dystonia or CP be given a trial of L-DOPA [39]. L-DOPA may be helpful in some children, even those with secondary dystonia [40].

Anticholinergic medication is very effective in acute dystonic reactions. It is partly effective in a subset of children with chronic dystonia [37]. Its mechanism of action for dystonia is not known, although it is presumed to have an effect on the large cholinergic interneurons of the striatum.

Diazepam and other benzodiazepines or sedative medications can occasionally be helpful. Baclofen has been used and may be effective in some cases, although its mechanism of effectiveness in dystonia is not known. Intrathecal baclofen can reduce tone in generalized dystonia if the catheter is placed at a cervical level [35]. Orthopedic procedures may not have expected outcomes in children with dystonia, as there is a tendency for dystonia to transfer to other muscles following an orthopedic procedure [2].

Neuromuscular Blocking Agents

When dystonia is associated with increased tone, botulinum toxin has been shown to be very effective in directly reducing the tone in the hypertonic muscles, but it may also be effective in changing the overall pattern of dystonia. In particular, it is sometimes observed that botulinum toxin injection into one muscle will relax other muscles of the same limb [41]. Botulinum toxin causes reversible denervation of the neuromuscular junction, due to the inhibition of the release of acetylcholine into the neuromuscular junction [77].

Neurosurgery

Neurosurgical intervention is reserved for the most severe cases, but the possibility that earlier surgical intervention may slow progression of the disease or lead to a longer disease-free interval has been raised. Pallidotomy and thalamotomy have been in use for many years, with some success.

More recently, deep brain stimulation has become available, and multiple targets have been attempted, including the ventrolateral thalamus. The advantage of deep brain stimulation is the ability to control the current delivery and the ability to select one or a combination of up to four electrodes through an external programmer. The stimulation wire is implanted using a combination of stereotactic neurosurgical techniques and usually microelectrode recording for precise localization. The lead is connected to a pacemaker implanted in the chest. For generalized dystonia, both sides usually need to be implanted [2].

Physical Therapy

Dystonia is a devastating neurological condition that prevents the acquisition of normal motor skills during critical periods of development in children [78]. In childhood dystonia, the ability to appropriately suppress variable and uncorrelated elements of movement is impaired [79]. Increased variability may represent an inability to suppress motor noise, resulting in the superposition of unwanted motion components on the desired movement. This may lead to more variable and less efficient motor outcomes, which are typical in dystonia. Muscle activity in dystonia typically exhibits both overflow into task-unrelated muscles and greater variability within task-related muscles than in healthy subjects [80–82].

A recent study showed that children with dystonic CP may benefit from physical therapy that specifically accommodates the unique motor control disorder [83]. Dystonia may not be a velocity-dependent hypersensitivity of reflexes and may include position-dependent muscle reflexes and co-contractions. Therefore, the correct positioning is essential to optimize vestibular responses and improve postural control [83].

Postural Reeducation

Stretching and strengthening of muscles can minimize physical limitations, prevent contractures and increase postural stability [77, 84–87], resulting in a decreased need for doses of botulinum toxin [85, 88]. Postural reeducation and soft tissue mobilization may reduce the pain in patients with cervical dystonia [84, 85].

Voos et al. [89] and Queiroz et al. [90] showed that exercises for the trunk, following the same principles of stretching shortened muscles, strengthening weak muscles, and stabilizing joints reduced pain and improved functional independence. Manual soft-tissue mobilization reduced local pain and discomfort and increased the passive range of motion [84, 85, 89, 90]. Smania et al. [84] , Tassorelli et al. [88] , and Ramdharry [85] observed that posture training reduced pain and improved functional performance in activities of daily living.

Constraint-Induced Movement Therapy

Constraint-induced movement therapy has been successfully used for the treatment of focal hand dystonia. Casting can decrease hand dystonia in patients with early onset, mild dystonia [91, 92]. However, the constraint must be used with caution as dystonia can worsen in a casted limb, and high forces incurred against the cast or brace may lead to skin breakdown.

Biofeedback

Several studies have reported positive effects of biofeedback of muscle activity in reducing muscle activation in individuals with dyskinetic CP. Two recent studies investigated the effectiveness of visual biofeedback of hand muscle activity in children with dystonia [93, 94]. Children with dystonia significantly reduced their co-contraction, in addition to their overflow of the nontask muscle activity when visual feedback was provided. These results indicate that children with dystonia are at least partially able to control co-contraction and reduce overflow.

A study of 10 children with dystonia reported significant improvement in arm function after using electromyography (EMG) biofeedback for 5 h per day for 1 month [95]. The mechanism of motor improvement using EMG biofeedback could be related to increased attention and enhanced sensation of muscle contraction mimicking proprioception. Another possible mechanism for improvement is the induction of plasticity associated with the increased correlation between a motor action and its sensory result. By increasing the sensation associated with muscle contraction, biofeedback can further enhance cortical or subcortical representations of movement [96].

Sensory Tricks

To deal with the dystonic movements, patients commonly adopt specific gestures, called "sensory tricks" [77]. Almost 90 % of patients report that sensory tricks (e.g., touching the chin, touching the posterior or superior part of the head) temporarily reduce involuntary movements [97, 98].

The increase in dystonic movements during motor activities (e.g., walking or writing) can be explained by a limitation of the central processing, which prevents the inhibition of dystonic movements during dual or multiple tasks. The decrease in these involuntary movements and improved control with sensory tricks may occur because of extra feedback provided by performing these strategies [87, 97]. The fact that some patients present a reduction in involuntary movements just by imagining that they were performing the sensory trick [99] suggests the occurrence of an important central modulation of the dystonic movements.

Sensory tricks are an important therapeutic strategy and can be used by physical therapists to gain functional independence and reduce discomfort. Crowner [87] proposed the use of sensory tricks during physical therapy to optimize functional gains, but mentioned that very few studies had tried this approach so far. Ramdharry [85] used a sensory cue (a light touch on the face) to help the patient to control dystonic muscles.

Kinesiotape

Kinesiotape may be an adjunct intervention to exercise, because kinesiotape enhances the patient's ability to control dystonic movements [89, 100]. According to Jankovic [86], external resources for providing better alignment may increase the proprioceptive feedback, helping the patient to develop sensory tricks and recruit antagonists of the dystonic pattern.

References

1. Blackburn JS, Mink JW, Augustine EF. Pediatric movement disorders: five new things. Neurol Clin Pract. 2012;2(4):311–18.
2. Sanger TD, Mink JW. Movement disorders. In: Swaiman KF, Ashwal S, Ferriero DM, Schor NF, editors. Swaiman's pediatric neurology. Philadelphia: Elsevier Saunders; 2012. p. 965–98.
3. Sanger TD, Chen D, Delgado MR, Gaebler-Spira D, Hallett M, Mink JW, et al. Definition and classification of negative motor signs in childhood. Pediatrics. 2006;118(5):2159–67.
4. Sanger TD, Chen D, Fehlings DL, Hallett M, Lang AE, Mink JW, et al. Definition and classification of hyperkinetic movements in childhood. Mov Disord. 2010;25(11):1538–49.
5. Sanger TD, Delgado MR, Gaebler-Spira D, Hallett M, Mink JW. Task force on childhood motor D. Classification and definition of disorders causing hypertonia in childhood. Pediatrics. 2003;111(1):e89–97.
6. Aicardi J, Bax M, Gillberg C. Diseases of the nervous system in childhood. 3rd ed. London: Mac Keith Press; 2009. p. 963.
7. Bax M, Goldstein M, Rosenbaum P, Leviton A, Paneth N, Dan B, et al. Proposed definition and classification of cerebral palsy, April 2005. Dev Med Child Neurol. 2005;47(8):571–6.
8. Swaiman KF, Wu YW. Cerebral palsy. In: Swaiman KF, Ashwal S, Ferriero DM, Schor NF, editors. Swaiman's pediatric neurology. Philadelphia: Elsevier Saunders; 2012. p. 999–1008.
9. Shevell MI, Dagenais L, Hall N, Consortium R. Comorbidities in cerebral palsy and their relationship to neurologic subtype and GMFCS level. Neurology. 2009;72(24):2090–6.
10. Ashwal S, Russman BS, Blasco PA, Miller G, Sandler A, Shevell M, et al. Practice parameter: diagnostic assessment of the child with cerebral palsy: report of the quality standards subcommittee of the American academy of neurology and the practice committee of the child neurology society. Neurology. 2004;62(6):851–63.
11. Rankin J, Cans C, Garne E, Colver A, Dolk H, Uldall P, et al. Congenital anomalies in children with cerebral palsy: a population-based record linkage study. Dev Med Child Neurol. 2010;52(4):345–51.
12. Cans C, Surman G, McManus V, Coghlan D, Hensey O, Johnson A. Cerebral palsy registries. Semin Pediatr Neurol. 2004;11(1):18–23.
13. Hagberg B, Hagberg G, Beckung E, Uvebrant P. Changing panorama of cerebral palsy in Sweden. VIII. Prevalence and origin in the birth year period 1991–94. Acta Paediatr. 2001;90(3):271–7.
14. Surveillance of Cerebral Palsy in Europe. Surveillance of cerebral palsy in Europe: a collaboration of cerebral palsy surveys and registers. Surveillance of cerebral palsy in Europe (SCPE). Dev Med Child Neurol. 2000;42(12):816–24.
15. McDonald AD. Cerebral palsy in children of very low birth weight. Arch Dis Child. 1963;38:579–88.
16. Hagberg B, Hagberg G, Zetterstrom R. Decreasing perinatal mortality—increase in cerebral palsy morbidity. Acta Paediatr Scand. 1989;78(5):664–70.
17. Scher MS, Dobson V, Carpenter NA, Guthrie RD. Visual and neurological outcome of infants with periventricular leukomalacia. Dev Med Child Neurol. 1989;31(3):353–65.
18. Chutorian AM, Michener RC, Defendini R, Hilal SK, Gamboa ET. Neonatal polycystic encephalomalacia: four new cases and review of the literature. J Neurol Neurosurg Psychiatry. 1979;42(2):154–60.
19. Lyen KR, Lingam S, Butterfill AM, Marshall WC, Dobbing CJ, Lee DS. Multicystic encephalomalacia due to fetal viral encephalitis. Eur J Pediatr. 1981;137(1):11–6.

20. Lynch JK. Epidemiology and classification of perinatal stroke. Semin Fetal Neonatal Med. 2009;14(5):245–9.
21. Himmelmann K, Hagberg G, Uvebrant P. The changing panorama of cerebral palsy in Sweden. X. Prevalence and origin in the birth-year period 1999–2002. Acta Paediatr. 2010;99(9):1337–43.
22. Bax M, Tydeman C, Flodmark O. Clinical and MRI correlates of cerebral palsy: the European Cerebral Palsy Study. JAMA. 2006;296(13):1602–8.
23. Uvebrant P. Hemiplegic cerebral palsy. Aetiology and outcome. Acta Paediatr Scand Suppl. 1988;345:1–100.
24. Wiklund LM, Uvebrant P, Flodmark O. Morphology of cerebral lesions in children with congenital hemiplegia. A study with computed tomography. Neuroradiology. 1990;32(3):179–86.
25. Black PD. Ocular defects in children with cerebral palsy. Br Med J. 1980;281(6238):487–8.
26. Brown JK, van Rensburg F, Walsh G, Lakie M, Wright GW. A neurological study of hand function of hemiplegic children. Dev Med Child Neurol. 1987;29(3):287–304.
27. Kyllerman M, Bager B, Bensch J, Bille B, Olow I, Voss H. Dyskinetic cerebral palsy. I. Clinical categories, associated neurological abnormalities and incidences. Acta Paediatr Scand. 1982;71(4):543–50.
28. Foley J. Dyskinetic and dystonic cerebral palsy and birth. Acta Paediatr. 1992;81(1):57–60. discussion 93–4.
29. Steinlin M, Zangger B, Boltshauser E. Non-progressive congenital ataxia with or without cerebellar hypoplasia: a review of 34 subjects. Dev Med Child Neurol. 1998;40(3):148–54.
30. Ferre C, Brandão M, Hung Y, Carmel J, Gordon A. Feasibility of caregiver-directed home-based hand-arm bimanual intensive training: a brief report. Dev Neurorehabil. 2015;18(1):69–74.
31. Shin JW, Song GB, Hwangbo G. Effects of conventional neurological treatment and a virtual reality training program on eye-hand coordination in children with cerebral palsy. J Phys Ther Sci. 2015;27(7):2151–4.
32. Thompson AM, Chow S, Vey C, Lloyd M. Constraint-induced movement therapy in children aged 5 to 9 years with cerebral palsy: a day camp model. Pediatr Phys Ther. 2015;27(1):72–80.
33. Merrill DR. Review of electrical stimulation in cerebral palsy and recommendations for future directions. Dev Med Child Neurol. 2009;51 Suppl 4:154–65.
34. Chiu HC, Ada L. Effect of functional electrical stimulation on activity in children with cerebral palsy: a systematic review. Pediatr Phys Ther. 2014;26(3):283–8.
35. Gannotti ME, Fuchs RK, Roberts DE, Hobbs N, Cannon IM. Health benefits of seated speed, resistance, and power training for an individual with spastic quadriplegic cerebral palsy: a case report. J Pediatr Rehabil Med. 2015;8(3):251–7.
36. Lee M, Ko Y, Shin MM, Lee W. The effects of progressive functional training on lower limb muscle architecture and motor function in children with spastic cerebral palsy. J Phys Ther Sci. 2015;27(5):1581–4.
37. Kim JH, Seo HJ. Effects of trunk-hip strengthening on standing in children with spastic diplegia: a comparative pilot study. J Phys Ther Sci. 2015;27(5):1337–40.
38. Franki I, Desloovere K, De Cat J, Tijhuis W, Molenaers G, Feys H, Vanderstraeten G, Van Den Broeck C. An evaluator-blinded randomized controlled trial evaluating therapy effects and prognostic factors for a general and an individually defined physical therapy program in ambulant children with bilateral spastic cerebral palsy. Eur J Phys Rehabil Med. 2015;51(6):677–91.
39. Abd El-Kafy EM, El-Basatiny HMYM. Effect of postural balance training on gait parameters in children with cerebral palsy. Am J Phys Med Rehabil. 2014;93:938–47.
40. Encheff JL, Armstrong C, Masterson M, et al. Hippotherapy effects on trunk, pelvic, and hip motion during ambulation in children with neurological impairments. Pediatr Phys Ther. 2012;24:242–50.
41. Pin T, Dyke P, Chan M. The effectiveness of passive stretching in children with cerebral palsy. Dev Med Child Neurol. 2006;48:855–62.
42. Richards CL, Malouin F, Dumas F. Effects of a single session of prolonged plantarflexor stretch on muscle activations during gait in spastic cerebral palsy. Scand J Rehabil Med. 1991;23:103–11.

43. Macias-Merlo L, Bagur-Calafat C, Girabent-Farrés M, Stuberg WA. Standing programs to promote hip flexibility in children with spastic diplegic cerebral palsy. Pediatr Phys Ther. 2015;27(3):243–9.
44. Macias-Merlo L, Bagur-Calafat C, Girabent-Farrés M, Stuberg WA. Effects of the standing program with hip abduction on hip acetabular development in children with spastic diplegia cerebral palsy. Disabil Rehabil. 2016;38(11):1075–81.
45. Yonetsu R, Iwata A, Surya J, Unase K, Shimizu J. Sit-to-stand movement changes in preschool-aged children with spastic diplegia following one neurodevelopmental treatment session—a pilot study. Disabil Rehabil. 2015;37(18):1643–50.
46. Cho C, Hwang W, Hwang S, Chung Y. Treadmill training with virtual reality improves gait, balance, and muscle strength in children with cerebral palsy. Tohoku J Exp Med. 2016;238(3):213–18.
47. Angsupaisal M, Visser B, Alkema A, Meinsma-van der Tuin M, Maathuis CG, Reinders-Messelink H, Hadders-Algra M. Therapist-designed adaptive riding in children with cerebral palsy: results of a feasibility study. Phys Ther. 2015;95(8):1151–62.
48. Flett PJ. Rehabilitation of spasticity and related problems in childhood cerebral palsy. J Paediatr Child Health. 2003;39:6–14.
49. AlSaif AA, Alsenany S. Effects of interactive games on motor performance in children with spastic cerebral palsy. J Phys Ther Sci. 2015;27(6):2001–3.
50. Kruijsen-Terpstra AJ, Verschuren O, Ketelaar M, Riedijk L, Gorter JW, Jongmans MJ, Boeije H. Parents' experiences and needs regarding physical and occupational therapy for their young children with cerebral palsy. Res Dev Disabil. 2016;53–54:314–22.
51. Remijn L, Speyer R, Groen BE, Holtus PC, van Limbeek J. Nijhuis-van der Sanden MW. Assessment of mastication in healthy children and children with cerebral palsy: a validity and consistency study. J Oral Rehabil. 2013;40(5):336–47.
52. Watson RM, Pennington L. Assessment and management of the communication difficulties of children with cerebral palsy: a UK survey of SLT practice. Int J Lang Commun Disord. 2015;50(2):241–59.
53. Heathcock JC, Baranet K, Ferrante R, Hendershot S. Daily intervention for young children with cerebral palsy in GMFCS level V: a case series. Pediatr Phys Ther. 2015;27(3):285–92.
54. Parry TS. The effectiveness of early intervention: a critical review. J Paediatr Child Health. 1992;28(5):343–6.
55. Lee SH, Shim JS, Kim K, Moon J, Kim M. Gross motor function outcome after intensive rehabilitation in children with bilateral spastic cerebral palsy. Ann Rehabil Med. 2015;39(4):624–9.
56. Palisano R, Rosenbaum P, Walter S, Russell D, Wood E, Galuppi B. Development and reliability of a system to classify gross motor function in children with cerebral palsy. Dev Med Child Neurol. 1997;39(4):214–23.
57. Hayley SM, Coster WI, Kao YC, Dumas HM, Fragala MA, Kramer JM, Ludlow LW, Moed R. Lessons from use of the PEDI: where do we go from where? Pediatr Phys Ther. 2010;22(1):69–75.
58. Styer-Acevedo J. Physical therapy for children with cerebral palsy. In: Tecklin J, editor. Pediatric Physical Therapy, 3rd edn. Artmed.
59. Bobath K, Bobath B. The neurodevelopmental treatment. In: Scrutton D, editor. Management of the motor disorders of children with cerebral palsy. Philadelphia: JB Lippincott; 1984. p. 6–18.
60. Temcharoensuk P, Lekskulchai R, Akamanon C, Ritruechai P, Sutcharitpongsa S. Effect of horseback riding versus a dynamic and static horse riding simulator on sitting ability of children with cerebral palsy: a randomized controlled trial. J Phys Ther Sci. 2015;27(1):273–7.
61. Park ES, Rha DW, Shin JS, Kim S, Jung S. Effects of hippotherapy on gross motor function and functional performance of children with cerebral palsy. Yonsei Med J. 2014;55(6):1736–42.
62. Lai CJ, Liu WY, Yang TF, Chen CL, Wu CY, Chan RC. Pediatric aquatic therapy on motor function and enjoyment in children diagnosed with cerebral palsy of various motor severities. J Child Neurol. 2015;30(2):200–8.

63. Radtka SA, Skinner SR, Johanson ME. A comparison of gait with solid and hinged ankle-foot orthoses in children with spastic diplegic cerebral palsy. Gait Posture. 1995;21(3):301–10.
64. Ries AJ, Novacheck TF, Schwartz MH. The efficacy of ankle-foot orthoses on improving the gait of children with diplegic cerebral palsy: a multiple outcome analysis. PM R. 2015;7(9):922–9.
65. Pranzatelli MR. Oral pharmacotherapy for the movement disorders of cerebral palsy. J Child Neurol. 1996;11 Suppl 1:S13–22.
66. Singer HS, Mink JW, Gilbert DL, Jankovic J. Cerebral palsy. In: Singer HS, Mink JW, Gilbert DL, Jankovic J, editors. Cerebral palsy. Philadelphia: Saunders; 2010. p. 2–8.
67. Simpson DM, Gracies JM, Graham HK, Miyasaki JM, Naumann M, Russman B, et al. Assessment: botulinum neurotoxin for the treatment of spasticity (an evidence-based review): report of the therapeutics and technology assessment subcommittee of the American academy of neurology. Neurology. 2008;70(19):1691–8.
68. Gilmartin R, Bruce D, Storrs BB, Abbott R, Krach L, Ward J, et al. Intrathecal baclofen for management of spastic cerebral palsy: multicenter trial. J Child Neurol. 2000;15(2):71–7.
69. Butler C, Campbell S. Evidence of the effects of intrathecal baclofen for spastic and dystonic cerebral palsy. AACPDM treatment outcomes committee review panel. Dev Med Child Neurol. 2000;42(9):634–45.
70. Fabry G, Liu XC, Molenaers G. Gait pattern in patients with spastic diplegic cerebral palsy who underwent staged operations. J Pediatr Orthop B. 1999;8(1):33–8.
71. Hoon Jr AH, Freese PO, Reinhardt EM, Wilson MA, Lawrie Jr WT, Harryman SE, et al. Age-dependent effects of trihexyphenidyl in extrapyramidal cerebral palsy. Pediatr Neurol. 2001;25(1):55–8.
72. Vidailhet M, Yelnik J, Lagrange C, Fraix V, Grabli D, Thobois S, et al. Bilateral pallidal deep brain stimulation for the treatment of patients with dystonia-choreoathetosis cerebral palsy: a prospective pilot study. Lancet Neurol. 2009;8(8):709–17.
73. Jethwa A, Mink J, Macarthur C, Knights S, Fehlings T, Fehlings D. Development of the hypertonia assessment tool (HAT): a discriminative tool for hypertonia in children. Dev Med Child Neurol. 2010;52(5):e83–7.
74. Burke RE, Fahn S, Marsden CD, Bressman SB, Moskowitz C, Friedman J. Validity and reliability of a rating scale for the primary torsion dystonias. Neurology. 1985;35:73–7.
75. Barry MJ, Van Swearingen JM, Albright AL. Reliability and responsiveness of the Barry-Albright dystonia scale. Dev Med Child Neurol. 1999;41:404–11.
76. Comella CL, Leurgans S, Wuu J, Stebbins GT, Chmura T. Dystonia study group. Rating scales for dystonia: a multicenter assessment. Mov Disord. 2003;18(3):303–12.
77. Tarsy D, Simon PK. Dystonia. N Engl J Med. 2006;8:818–29.
78. Bertucco M, Sanger TD. Current and emerging strategies for treatment of childhood dystonia. J Hand Ther. 2015;28(2):185–93.
79. Lunardini F, Maggioni S, Casellato C, Bertucco M, Pedrocchi AL, Sanger TD. Increased task-uncorrelated muscle activity in childhood dystonia. J Neuroeng Rehabil. 2015;12:52.
80. Bertucco M, Sanger TD. Speed-accuracy testing on the Apple iPad® provides a quantitative test of upper extremity motor performance in children with dystonia. J Child Neurol. 2014;29:1460–6.
81. Casellato C, Maggioni S, Lunardini F, Bertucco M, Pedrocchi A, Sanger TD. Dystonia: altered sensorimotor control and vibro-tactile EMG-based biofeedback effects. XIII Mediterranean Conference on Medical and Biological Engineering and Computing 2013 IFMBE Proceedings; p. 1742–46.
82. Chu WTV, Sanger TD. Force variability during isometric biceps contraction in children with secondary dystonia due to cerebral palsy. Mov Disord. 2009;24:1299–305.
83. Androwis GJ, Michael PA, Jewaid D, Nolan KJ, Strongwater A, Foulds RA. Motor control investigation of dystonic cerebral palsy: a pilot study of passive knee trajectory. Conf Proc IEEE Eng Med Biol Soc. 2015;2015:4562–5.

84. Smania N, Corato E, Tinazzi M, Montagnana B, Fiaschi A, Aglioti SM. The effect of two different rehabilitation treatments in cervical dystonia: preliminary results in four patients. Funct Neurol. 2003;4:219–25.
85. Ramdharry G. Case report: physiotherapy cuts the dose of botulinum toxin. Physiother Res Int. 2006;2:117–22.
86. Jankovic J. Treatment of dystonia. Lancet Neurol. 2006;5:864–72.
87. Crowner BE. Cervical dystonia: disease profile and clinical management. Phys Ther. 2007;11:1511–26.
88. Tassorelli C, Mancini F, Balloni L, Pacchetti C, Sandrini G, Nappi G, Martignoni E. Botulinum toxin and neuromotor rehabilitation: an integrated approach to idiopathic cervical dystonia. Mov Disord. 2006;12:2240–3.
89. Voos MC, Oliveira TP, Piemonte MEP, Barbosa ER. Case report: physical therapy management of axial dystonia. Physiother Theory Pract. 2014;30(1):56–61.
90. Queiroz MA, Chien HF, Sekeff-Sallem FA, Barbosa ER. Physical therapy program for cervical dystonia: a study of 20 cases. Funct Neurol. 2012;27:187–92.
91. Pesenti A, Barbieri S, Priori A. Limb immobilization for occupational dystonia: a possible alternative treatment for selected patients. Adv Neurol. 2004;94:247–54.
92. Priori A, Pesenti A, Cappellari A, Scarlato G, Barbieri S. Limb immobilization for the treatment of focal occupational dystonia. Neurology. 2001;57:405–9.
93. Young SJ, van Doornik J, Sanger TD. Finger muscle control in children with dystonia. Mov Disord. 2011;26(7):1290–6.
94. Young SJ, van Doornik J, Sanger TD. Visual feedback reduces co-contraction in children with dystonia. J Child Neurol. 2011;26(1):37–43.
95. Bloom R, Przekop A, Sanger TD. Prolonged electromyogram biofeedback improves upper extremity function in children with cerebral palsy. J Child Neurol. 2010;25(12):1480–4.
96. Casellato C, Zorzi G, Pedrocchi A, Ferrigno G, Nardocci N. Reaching and writing movements: sensitive and reliable tools to measure genetic dystonia in children. J Child Neurol. 2011;26:822–9.
97. Jahanshahi M. Factors that ameliorate or aggravate spasmodic torticollis. J Neurol Neurosurg Psychiatry. 2000;2:227–9.
98. Schramm A, Reiners K, Naumann M. Complex mechanisms of sensory tricks in cervical dystonia. Mov Disord. 2004;4:452–8.
99. Bressman SB. Dystonia genotypes, phenotypes, and classification. Adv Neurol. 2004;94:101–7.
100. Kase K, Tatsuyuki H, Tomoki O. Kinesio taping perfect manual. Kinesio Taping Assoc. 1996;6:117–18.

Future Perspectives: Assessment Tools and Rehabilitation in the New Age

10

Greydon Gilmore and Mandar Jog

Abbreviations

BG   Basal ganglia
FOG   Freezing of gait
IRED   Infrared-emitting diode
LED   Light-emitting diode
MD   Movement disorder
PD   Parkinson's disease
UPDRS   Unified Parkinson's Disease Rating Scale
VR   Virtual reality

Introduction

The clinical study of movement disorders (MDs) remains a challenge, despite the advancement of technology, stemming partially from the difficulty of objectively studying the effect of the disease and its impact on the physical and mental state of the patient. Currently, validated methods for such assessments are entirely scale-based and hence face the issues of intra- and inter-rater reliability, correlation with the aspects of quality of life that actually affect the patient, and additionally, are not particularly sensitive to the therapeutic interventions that exist for these diseases.

G. Gilmore, M.Sc., B.Sc.
Physiology and Pharmacology, Western University,
London, ON, Canada N6A 3K7
e-mail: greydon.gilmore@gmail.com

M. Jog, M.D., F.R.C.P.C. (✉)
Clinical Neurological Sciences, London Health Sciences Centre,
London, ON, Canada N6A 5A5
e-mail: mandar.jog@lhsc.on.ca

© Springer International Publishing Switzerland 2017   155
H.F. Chien, O.G.P. Barsottini (eds.), *Movement Disorders Rehabilitation*,
DOI 10.1007/978-3-319-46062-8_10

The use of objective measurements for titration and adjustment of therapy is well accepted in disorders such as hypertension and diabetes. Medical management of these conditions is critically dependent on the measurement of the individual variables, namely blood pressure and blood sugar. At present, no such technique is being used in the clinical treatment of neurodegenerative disorders. Researchers have improved the reliability of disease assessment ratings through the increased use of objective and quantitative data collection tools over the past few years [1]. A recent review discussed current technology and the potential for these technologies to replace outdated clinical rating scales [1]. The advancement of successful and established (e.g., levodopa for Parkinson's disease) in addition to more complex interventions (e.g., deep brain stimulation, Duodopa pump treatment) has accentuated the need for improved assessment measures for many disorders. The question of "man versus machine," increasing the use of technology to counter subjectivity, has become more prevalent in the current literature looking to assess and quantify patient symptom profiles [1]. The primary goal of these attempts is to provide the clinician with a useful and noncumbersome yet reliable tool kit, especially for issues regarding mobility, to adjust therapy and thereby improve the patient's quality of life.

Parkinson's disease (PD) is a neurodegenerative MD presenting with several common hallmark motor symptoms such as: tremor, bradykinesia, dyskinesia, balance difficulty, falls, and gait impairment [5]. The primary pathophysiological cause of the PD motor symptomatology is the neurodegeneration of dopaminergic neurons in the substantia nigra pars compacta (SNc) within the basal ganglia (BG) [5]. One of the key features of the PD motor symptoms is that they manifest when there is a 60–80 % loss of dopaminergic neurons within the SNc [5]. PD is complicated further by frequently observed comorbid nonmotor symptoms, such as depression, cognitive deficits and sleep disturbances [5]. The nonmotor symptoms arise, in part, from neurodegeneration within other areas, including the cortex and locus ceruleus [5]. The important point here is that this spectrum of motor and nonmotor symptoms varies from person to person, and tends to become increasingly fluctuant as the disease progresses, requiring highly individualized therapy. In this chapter, PD is used as the signature disease to address the concepts of technology-based mobility assessment and individualized treatment optimization/rehabilitation.

To provide such individualized therapy, patients are currently required to meet with the physician in clinic every 6 months to a year, for a short period of time. The clinic visit provides a snapshot of the patient's condition, which often does not reflect the daily challenges that the patient may face and the assessment tools are not adequate to provide an insight into this issue. Given the lack of such measures (except for subjective quality of life scales), the clinician finds it virtually impossible to titrate management, medical, surgical or rehabilitative, to actually improve such function. Indeed, the adjustment of therapy is largely directed at the subjective reporting of the motor state and the observed motor state, but not during the performance of functional tasks. Furthermore, in clinical practice severity evaluation and adjustments in treatment rely too heavily on the clinicians' expertise, which lacks inter-rater reliability [1, 10]. The use of more objective and quantitative motor assessment methods, carried out while the patient is performing some standardized activity of daily living tasks, which can then be used to optimize medical and rehabilitative management, is imperative in improving the quality of life for individuals diagnosed with PD. Although this approach is not likely to change the course of the disease, it may allow the patient with PD to continue to experience some control of their autonomy while dealing with increasing disease disability.

Clark [11] first proposed the concept of physical therapy as a treatment option for PD, even before the implementation of levodopa in the 1960s by Birkmayer [11]. Clark [11] described implementing specific exercises to help to improve the speed of extremities and to maintain these exercises to "prevent the deleterious effects of inactivity." Currently, rehabilitation is considered an effective adjunctive therapy to pharmaceutical and surgical treatments. Physical therapy rehabilitation allows for the maximization of functional abilities and improved quality of life. However, until recently, the underlying mechanism was unknown. The physical therapy rehabilitation techniques currently used are not suitable for individuals with PD owing to the symptomatic constraints of the disease. A recent meta-analysis examined current physical therapy techniques in individuals with PD and found that it provides only a transient improvement of motor symptoms [11]. Another randomized clinical trial explored the clinical effectiveness of individualized physiotherapy in a population of 762 individuals with PD [11]. It was found that physiotherapy was not associated with immediate clinically meaningful improvements in mild and moderate PD [11]. A successful rehabilitation technique for individuals with PD requires ecologically valid tasks that these individuals would normally perform every day. Furthermore, the area where the training occurs should be suitable for each patient as individuals may perform better in their own home or environments closer to home than in a clinic. Most importantly, rehabilitative techniques are often not available except at specialized centers requiring travel which is a difficult and unmanageable venture for most patients and caregivers. Hence, another way of bringing practical yet specialized rehabilitation techniques, i.e., those that are smart and portable, close to the patient, is a significant unmet need.

The assessment, treatment, and rehabilitation of PD are all interrelated and require integration in a potentially seamless manner to provide treatment optimization and thereby improve the quality of life for these individuals. This chapter explores the up and coming assessment, treatment, and rehabilitation techniques that are currently being explored for application in individuals with PD as one such scenario of a new frontier. Laboratory-based technologies in addition to portable and wearable systems for mobility assessment are discussed. Finally, a new methodology based on virtual reality (VR) for generating real-world scenarios within which patients can be assessed for medical management optimization and potentially for providing portable and targeted rehabilitation is explored.

In summary, the current needs of rehabilitation for PD are:

1. Subjective measures for recording physical/motor disability that are currently performed using clinical scales need to be replaced by objective instrument-based techniques. Such techniques would be portable, repeatable, and standardized.

2. Rehabilitative interventions are nonspecific and do not take into account the type of deficits that these patients face, namely strategy in performing activities of daily living. This needs to change.
3. An intelligent rehabilitation program would therefore be individualized to the disease, the stage of disease, and the patient's own perceived disability.
4. Assessment of the disability would be carried out within such an environment and based upon the detected performance difficulty, a rehabilitative strategy would be implemented.

Currently Used Scale-Based Assessment Techniques

The clinical assessment and monitoring of PD is challenging partly because of the complexity and heterogeneity of the disease. The methods used rely heavily on the clinicians' experience, which is inherently subjective and qualitative. There are a few commonly used assessment and monitoring techniques such as clinical rating scales, patient self-report, and patient diaries.

Clinical scales are used during the patient's visit and provide a quick overview of the current disease status. The most common clinical rating scale for PD is the Unified Parkinson's Disease Rating Scale (UPDRS). The UPDRS is the current gold standard for assessing and monitoring PD symptom severity. Part II is a subjective scale that assesses the impact of some of the activities of daily living. Part III of the UPDRS is a 31-item section used to rate motor symptom severity [15]. More specifically, the UPDRS contains an integer rating scale (0–4) to assess severity. A rating of 0 would be normal whereas a rating of 4 would indicate severe disability.

This assessment approach has several weaknesses that may hinder proper clinical care. The limited scoring range of the UPDRS decreases the sensitivity of the scale to detect smaller symptom changes. The UPDRS maintains intrinsic subjectivity and low inter-rater reliability, which limit its value as a measure in clinical diagnosis and research [10]. Individuals with PD who have more advanced disease tend to have fluctuations in their motor symptoms. The UPDRS, performed in the clinic, provides only a "snap-shot" of these fluctuations and may not reveal the true functional disability they experience while they are at home. In the context of this chapter, the main weakness of the scale is its inability to correlate Part II with Part III. That is, the functional impairment to the supposed activity of daily living due to the motor disability is not what is actually assessed during the motor examination. For example, the finger tapping task does not accurately reflect the ability to do up buttons, nor does the foot tapping task reflect leg mobility while standing or walking. In fact, the motor assessment is grossly incomplete and does not provide any resolution for important components such as balance, walking, and postural changes during goal-directed task performance. Therefore, how walking changes might affect a person going from a carpeted floor to tiles or the impact of turning in the kitchen during a cooking task, are not assessed. Indeed, the patient-driven part II and the clinician-performed part III do not give the clinician any reproducible way to titrate medical or surgical treatment. It certainly does not help to design a rehabilitation program that would target the deficits that the patient has identified in part II of the UPDRS. The clinician then targets part III while the expectation is that somehow, directly or indirectly, an improvement in this rating would automatically translate to an improvement in some aspects of part II.

Patient self-report and writing diary cards take place outside of clinic, usually in the patient's own home. The benefits of these techniques are that they can be completed in an environment in which the patient is comfortable and provide a more detailed perspective of how they are functioning. However, these methods are subjective and rely on the patient's understanding of their own symptoms. Self-report relies heavily on the patient recalling all symptoms experienced from memory. Introducing diary cards greatly enhances self-report. The many limitations of using diary cards, especially in patients that have motor and possibly some degree of cognitive deficit are obvious. Patient compliance, recall bias, and fatigue from diary writing are just some of the issues facing this method of recording the impact of PD-related motor disability on daily function. However, the most important issue in home-based assessments by the patients themselves regarding their function is the lack of an objective motor state of the patient. Therefore, although these methods may be somewhat more realistic in their ability to generate data that indicate real-world deficits, it is not paired with the much-needed objective clinical assessment. The gap and disconnect therefore continues to exist.

In summary, the scale-based assessment techniques currently used:

1. Are short and often not reflective of the patient's real-world experience of functional impairment
2. Often differ from what patients may be like in their own home compared with in clinic assessments
3. Hold an inherent disconnect between the disability perceived by patients during the performance of the activities of daily living (including those such as crossing the street, putting clothes in the washing machine, etc.) and the motor rating made by the clinician in the clinic
4. Are poor in their accuracy and the ones that may be more accurate are not carried out with a simultaneous motor assessment such as PD diaries and self-report
5. Lead to a state where management decisions are being made based largely on inaccurate and often nonrepresentative data, which reduces functional therapeutic optimization.

Current Technology-Based Assessment Techniques

Objective and quantitative monitoring of PD motor symptoms has the potential to address the unmet needs identified with the current scale based tools. They can provide a measurable and quantitative set of information of the current disease state. These measurements can be accurately taken serially and allow the assessment of the effectiveness of various therapeutic interventions. Accuracy of symptom measurement in individuals with PD is clinically imperative when deciding on treatment options and measuring their effect. Advancement in technology has provided the capability of monitoring human kinetics objectively and quantitatively. Various technology assessment tools have been developed and implemented for PD symptom monitoring. These assessment tools can either be laboratory-based or more portable for at-home use.

Laboratory-Based Methods

Vicon System

The Vicon™ system is an optical motion capture system that uses multiple cameras and body segment markers to capture body movements in 3D (Fig. 10.1a). Each Vicon camera is surrounded by a ring of light-emitting diodes (LEDs) that emit infra-red light (Fig. 10.1b). Infra-red reflective markers are attached to the individual on various body segments, the suggested number of markers to be used is 35–38 (Fig. 10.1c). As the participant walks in the capture zone the camera LEDs emit infra-red light that bounces off the body markers and is picked up by the Vicon

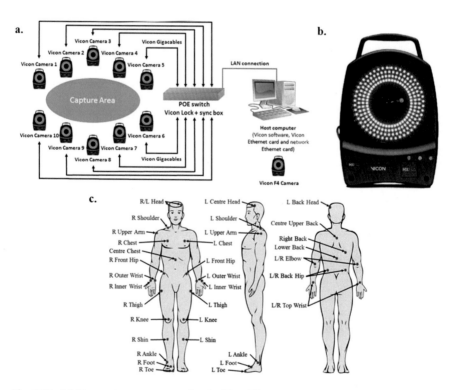

Fig. 10.1 (a) The measurement set up for the Vicon™ camera system. (b) The standard Vicon F40™ camera, reproduced with permission from MocapHouse [20]. (c) The standard infra-red reflective body marker positions required for accurate measurement [20]

Fig. 10.2   The Zeno™
walkway carpet system
used to monitor gait
performance in real time,
image provided courtesy of
Protokinetics

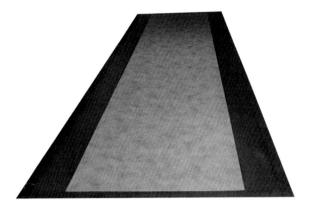

cameras. Each Vicon camera sends a 2D image to the MX Ultranet HD box every fraction of a second. The Ultranet box uses trigonometry to estimate the position of each marker in 3D; thus, each marker needs to be visible by at least two cameras at one time. The system is highly accurate and is able to detect movements within 1 mm at 250 frames per second [16, 17].

Das et al. [18] used the Vicon motion capture system in a population of individuals with PD and found a high correlation with the UPDRS. Many cardinal features of PD can be captured and analyzed using the proprietary software that is provided with this system. Such as tremor, bradykinesia, gait and postural stability [18]. Mirek et al. [18] explored the difference in gait parameter measures between PD and healthy control participants. It was found that the Vicon system was able to accurately detect a reduction in several gait measures in PD and control participants.

The main drawback to this system is the lack of portability. The system requires a large area for set-up and confines the individual to a round area where the cameras are able to record. If the individual moves outside the boundaries, the system will be unable to track their movements. The required number of body markers makes assessments with patients difficult because placing all the required markers is very time-consuming. The Vicon system is one of the more expensive motion capture technologies on the market, which limits the number of research laboratories that may be able to use it.

Gait Analysis Carpet System

Various gait assessment tools have been developed to quantify gait parameters while individuals walk across a pad with sensors. The Zeno walkway (Zenometrics™ LLC, Peekskill, NY, USA) is a 7-m-long carpet with embedded pressure sensors (Fig. 10.2). The sensors detect each footfall made by the participant while walking and relay the information to a computer for analysis. The software system captures each footfall on the Zeno walkway and provides accurate measurement of various spatial and temporal gait measures such as step length, stride velocity, single support time, double support time, and cadence, among many others [21, 22]. The sensor recording hardware is common to two main analysis software platforms,

GaitRite™ and PKMAS™. The validity and reliability of both software analysis systems has been shown in many studies to date [10, 23, 24]. Van Uden and Besser [24] examined the test–retest reliability of the Zeno walkway over a 1-week period. An intra-class correlation coefficient of over 0.90 was obtained for all spatial and temporal gait measures [24].

The Zeno walkway system allows the participant's gait performance to be quantified in an efficient manner, allowing post-hoc analysis to be conducted [4]. The ability to extract gait parameters during a patient's walk in real time has advanced the way in which treatment regimens are assessed. Obtaining these gait parameters can elucidate the characterization of disease [25, 26], the prediction of falls [27], and contribute to defining gait patterns in the progression of PD [28].

The main drawback to the Zeno walkway system is that it only provides 7 m of walking distance for analysis, which may not be a good representation of the general walking of the patient. Furthermore, a recent study examined the potential Hawthorne effect that arises while using the gait carpet [29]. It was found that patients walked significantly better when they knew they were being examined on the gait carpet [29]. The gait carpet system also needs to be used in a laboratory setting and is not a viable option for at-home monitoring.

In summary, laboratory based assessment techniques:

1. Are highly accurate and are able to record very reliably at a high resolution
2. Require the presence of a gait laboratory
3. Are not portable and need specialist expertise to be able to use
4. Are expensive and because of their very nature are primarily confined to academic institutions for gait and biomechanical research

Portable and Mobile Methods

Tele-monitoring is the remote monitoring of patients who are not at the same location as the health care provider. The ability of technology to provide a detailed objective and quantitative review of PD symptoms is making at-home monitoring a possibility. At-home assessment tools provide a method of observing patient symptoms on a continuous long-term basis. In this way, health care standards would improve and the cost would decrease. Patel et al. [30] developed a system that allowed tracking of PD motor fluctuations in the person's own home. The PD participants wore eight sensors that were connected to a web-based platform that sent data directly to the health care center. This system provided only details about motor fluctuations, but this method could be applied to other technologies to advance at-home monitoring of PD. Several of the systems currently available for home monitoring are reviewed briefly.

Kinect

The Kinect™ is a motion-sensing input device that provides full-body 3D motion capture (Fig. 10.3a). This system is used to directly control computer games through

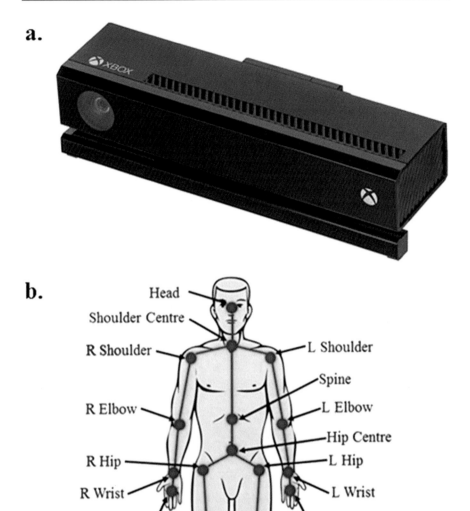

Fig. 10.3 (**a**) The standard Kinect™ system for Xbox One™ developed by Microsoft™, image from Wikimedia commons [32]. (**b**) The 20 key points that the Kinect sensor uses to generate a general skeleton for tracking users

body movement. One main strength of this system is that it is affordable and can be easily purchased. This system can be quickly set up anywhere and does not require markers to be placed on the body. Cancela et al. [31] developed a method for tracking gait performance in healthy subjects. They were able to track several features of the gait cycle with minimal error. Galna et al. [17] tested the Kinect system in 15 individuals diagnosed with PD. This group found that Kinect was able to track gross body segment movements very well, but fell short when attempting to track finer movements (such as toe tapping and tremor) [17]. Kinetic can currently be used to track bradykinesia quite well [17].

Currently, the system estimates the position of 20 anatomical landmarks (Fig. 10.3b). This estimation needs to be much more accurate and should have the capability to optimally adjust these landmarks for personalized use. The Kinect system is not portable, once it is set up the individual can only move a certain distance away and to the side of the sensor. However, this system is a viable option for at-home UPDRS assessment of patients. The patient can perform various motor assessment tasks in their own home while in front of the Kinect system.

Optotrak

Optotrak™ is a three-dimensional camera system used to track the motion of infrared emitting diode (IRED) markers (Fig. 10.4a). The IRED markers are placed on body segments of participants and the Optotrak camera tracks the movement of the markers in real time. The camera unit has a limited range within which participants have to stay for proper tracking (Fig. 10.4b). Optotrak has addressed this limitation and allows up to eight camera units to be used, which greatly expands the area of assessment. The Optotrak software provides kinematic data that are clinically relevant to individuals with PD, such as gait measures, tremor detection, and bradykinesia.

A recent study compared the gait measures extracted from the Optotrak system and the Kinect system. The agreement between the body measurements of the two systems was assessed using an intra-class correlation coefficient. It was found that gait parameters obtained from Kinect match well with the Optotrak system [31]. The Optotrak system is expensive, especially when acquiring more than one camera unit. The area of tracking for one camera unit is not sufficient for accurate body assessments and several units would need to be used for proper assessment. Although the Optotrak system has the advantage of being able to track finer movements, technology is quickly advancing and less expensive options may become available.

Wearable Inertial Sensors

Wearable inertial sensors are commonly used to measure motion and physical activity associated with daily living [34, 35]. The small size and ease of use make them ideal for placement on various body segments for real-time portable capture of multi-segmental body movements. The gaming and film industry has made use of these sensors in the design and development of their products. The clinical application of these sensors is still in its infancy but this application is quickly garnering attention.

a.

b.

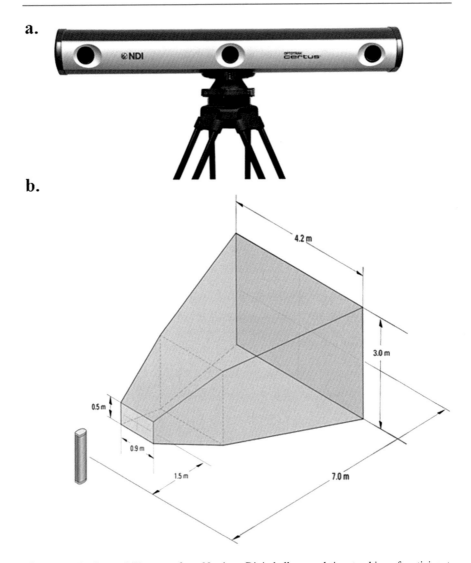

Fig. 10.4 The Optotrak™ system from Northern Digital allows real-time tracking of participants wearing infrared emitting diode markers. (**a**) The camera system used to track the markers, up to eight camera units can be used simultaneously, image provided courtesy of Northern Digital Inc. (**b**) The area of tracking for each camera unit, image provided courtesy of Northern Digital Inc.

There are three classes of inertial sensors. The combined signals of all three sensors have been used to accurately determine the temporal and spatial measures of body movement. The sensors are:

1. **Accelerometers**: measure the acceleration of linear motion. According to Newton's second law acceleration of linear motion is the force acting on a mass.

Accelerometers can be used to assess balance, gait and classification of movements.

2. **Gyroscopes**: measure the angular velocity giving information about orientation and rotation. These sensors allow recognition of movement within a 3D space.
3. **Magnetometers**: measure the precise movements of the body in the earth's magnetic field.

Wearable inertial sensors have been useful for application in assessing MDs [1, 36–38]. Chang et al. [39] developed a fall detection system by using three sensors (containing an accelerometer and gyroscope) placed on both feet and the waist. This study was able to accurately predict fall risk in various terrains including: motionless, walking, running, walking up an incline and climbing stairs [39].

Several studies have compared the UPDRS with the inertial sensors [40, 41]. Salarian et al. [41] found a high correlation between the total UPDRS and the data collected from three sensors in ten PD participants. This group was interested in monitoring ambulatory activity in a population of individuals with PD. PD often presents as an asymmetric disorder, one side of the body being more severely affected than the other. Sant'Anna et al. [40] assessed asymmetry of both lower and upper limbs during ambulation. The study used four sensors (both legs and wrists) to track asymmetry in 15 PD participants. They found a strong correlation (0.949) between the asymmetry scores of the UPDRS and the asymmetry values from the body sensors [40].

The inertial sensors are able to detect very fine movements, which patients and clinicians' do not notice. It is often argued that if patients do not notice the small changes in the parkinsonian state then employing these sensors is "overkill." However, this attribute could be beneficial for early diagnosis of PD by providing data that the clinical scales cannot detect [42]. Furthermore, the ability to detect such fine changes in the parkinsonian state may be beneficial in evaluating the efficacy of new treatments. These claims have to be validated in terms of making a difference in the diagnosis and treatment of patients. As such they remain predominantly in the research domain.

Kinesia

The Kinesia™ system (Cleveland Medical Devices Inc., Cleveland, OH, USA) is marketed as a clinical deployable technology that tracks tremor and bradykinesia in individuals with PD. This device is worn on a single finger, making the device very compact (Fig. 10.5). It has three accelerometers to track linear acceleration and three gyroscopes to measure angular velocity [43]. The device has shown test–retest reliability over clinic-based assessment techniques [44].

Motor symptoms of PD affect the entire body, which is a major concern with the Kinesia device. While it may be useful for detecting tremor and bradykinesia in the hand, it can provide limited detail about the symptom severity in the contralateral lower limb. Furthermore, PD motor symptoms are commonly asymmetric and affect one side more than the other [45, 46]. The motor symptoms may present bilaterally, but the severity of the symptoms may not be symmetrical [45]. The asymmetry of the disease represents another drawback for the Kinesia system.

Fig. 10.5 The Kinesia One™ sensor, which is placed on the fingertip and can monitor motor symptoms of PD, image provided courtesy of Kinesia

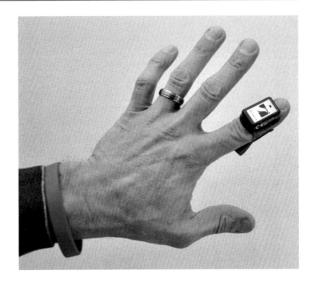

Motion Capture Suit

A full body sensor system is an appealing assessment technique that is gaining interest in the PD research field. Several motion capture suits have been used for research from animation companies such as Xsens™ and Synertial™ (Fig. 10.6a). These systems contain 16–19 inertial sensors that are located all over the body and provide information about all body segments (Fig. 10.6b). Research with the motion capture suit systems have shown reliability and validity at monitoring human movement [37, 47, 48]. These motion capture systems allow assessments to be completed outside of clinic and in the patients' own home environment.

Motion capture suit systems provide large quantities of data that need to be properly assessed for clinical impact. The main concern of these types of systems is the ability to extract relevant features. As previously mentioned, these sensors can detect small changes in body movements, but extracting these data for clinical application is not yet possible.

In summary, portable and mobile assessment methods:

1. Can be divided into those that are cheap and easy to implement but have lower resolution and those that provide very accurate information but large data sets.
2. Can be divided into sensor systems that utilize single or a small number of sensors for monitoring global body movements versus those that can monitor whole-body responses. To monitor single body parts (such as one limb) or to generate a global mobility score, single sensor systems may have some value. However, if a more detailed and whole-body measurement is required, then a multi-sensor system including body suit-type systems is more useful.
3. Are now becoming very affordable to buy, but lack the analysis software support to directly help clinicians to make management decisions.
4. Generally remain in the research domain, although vigorous efforts are on-going to make them clinically useful.

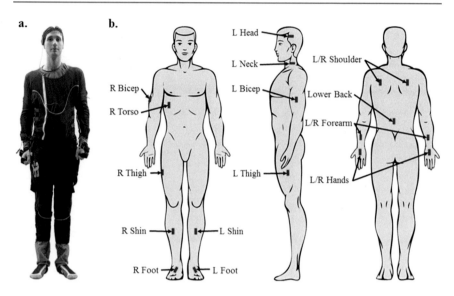

Fig. 10.6 The Synertial™ motion capture suit employs 17 sensors each containing a magnetometer, accelerometer, and gyroscope. The set-up time is minimal as the sensors are pre-placed onto the pants and top. (**a**) The Lycra motion capture, which houses 17 inertial sensors, reproduced with permission from LHSC [49]. (**b**) Diagram depicting the placement of the 17 inertial sensors on the body

Rehabilitation Approaches in Current Use

Despite optimal pharmacological treatment, the motor impairments in individuals with PD continue to deteriorate, leading to further impaired mobility [50]. The implementation of rehabilitation therapy is used as adjunctive treatment for troubling motor symptoms of PD. A multidisciplinary management plan for PD that incorporates both medical and rehabilitation therapy should be implemented to better manage the complex MD [51]. Medical management of PD is well understood. Additionally, several studies have shown supportive evidence for the implementation of rehabilitation techniques for PD management in combination [52]. Current rehabilitation techniques are discussed.

Rehabilitation Techniques for PD

Currently, physical therapy is the most widely used rehabilitation technique for the management of PD, focusing on improvements in gait, physical capacity (i.e., strength and endurance), posture, and balance [52]. Morris [53] was to our knowledge the first to describe a model of physical therapy management for individuals with PD. He proposed that the ability to move is not lost in PD; rather, it is an activation problem [53]. Morris suggested that the deficit in activation forces individuals with PD to rely on cortical control mechanisms to initiate movement [53]. The model used task-specific strategies such as gait, sitting down, and turning in bed.

The model made use of external cues such as visual, auditory, and proprioceptive stimuli (rocking the body from side to side) [53]. In a healthy human brain, the BG are related to the triggering of internal cues for performing a desired motor function [54, 55]. In PD, such internal cued movements may be significantly affected because of the complex cortical–basal ganglionic dysfunction [54, 56, 57]. It is also possible that these cues are not used to select and modify the required motor response correctly. The results may be seen as a disruption of normal motor function in appendicular and axial systems, including gait. In this context of PD, the external cues used allow alternative brain circuits to be recruited, bypassing the defective BG circuitry [54]. Verschueren et al. [56] studied the influence of extern— cues on motor task performance In a population of PD participants, who were trained to perform a motor task that provided external feedback during the performance of the task. The PD participants were then asked to complete the motor task while blindfolded, eliminating the external feedback. It was found that performance was significantly reduced in PD participants when performing the task blindfolded [56]. It was concluded that providing the external feedback during the performance phase allowed PD participants to partially bypass the BG [54, 56]. A recent review of literature highlighted this fact that external cues access alternative neural pathways that remain intact in the PD brain, such as the cerebello-thalamo-cortical network [58].

The ability to put together a temporal order of task performance is thus very difficult for patients with PD, leading to task failure or "freezing." Such difficulties can be seen in all aspects of motor performance. To address this, the training model discussed above also used cognitive movement strategies, which break complex movements into separate components [53]. Individuals with PD are trained to perform each component separately and to pay conscious attention to their execution. Morris [59] provided some updates to the physical therapy model focusing on adjusting the rehabilitation strategy based on years of diagnosis. Morris suggests that the tasks used in newly diagnosed individuals should be different from individuals who have been diagnosed for more than 5 years. This is because of the progressive death of substantia nigra cells, despite optimal pharmacological intervention [59].

A recent meta-analysis, conducted by Tomlinson et al. [13], examined the effectiveness of physical therapy in 33 randomized clinical trials with over 1,500 PD participants. Tomlinson et al. [13] found that physiotherapy intervention provides a transient benefit in the treatment of PD, regardless of the physiotherapy intervention. However, in the long term, benefit from physiotherapy remains elusive [13]. This meta-analysis states that an issue with current studies focused on physical therapy for PD is that outcome measures are drastically different [13]. They suggest employing relevant, reliable, and sensitive outcome measures, which hints at both measurement of the physical improvement using reliable tools (such as the systems mentioned above), but also functional improvements in the tasks that actually matter to the patient. Indeed, an improvement in the endurance or strength in a PD population may not matter to the performance of a task such as doing the laundry or crossing the street.

Another issue with current physical therapy models for PD stems from the symptomatic constraints in PD such as rigidity, bradykinesia, freezing, and impaired cognitive processing. Traditional rehabilitation techniques are not suitable for individuals with PD. King and Horak [60] developed an exercise program that was more suited to individuals with PD. However, the program was not adaptable to the various stages of the disease. A rehabilitation program, with functionally relevant tasks, that has direct applicability to the activities of daily living is a necessity. Providing a single space for rehabilitation for every patient is not ideal, as some patients may perform better in the contrived space [29]. Currently, PD patients are enrolled in standardized rehabilitation programs, in a contrived space, to carry out tasks that may not be applicable to their everyday life.

In summary, currently used rehabilitation techniques used for neurological diseases, especially PD:

1. Are nonspecific to the actual condition and stage of disease.
2. Are not targeted toward directly assessing and improving the functional impairments faced by the patient in daily life. Instead, nonspecific rehabilitation such as relaxation, stretching, cardiovascular fitness, and weight training are performed.
3. Could be more accurately assessed by using the sensor technologies discussed above to record out-of-laboratory mobility.
4. Are conducted in environments and contexts that are not yet individualized to the deficits of the disease.

Targeted, Disability-Based Rehabilitative Approaches to Parkinson's Disease

There are very few practical and useful devices available on the market for the specific treatment of PD symptoms. The two reviewed below are the only ones that have been adopted to some degree by patients and physicians. In the first instance, sensor technology is employed to measure a specific symptom, namely tremor, and a "made-to-measure" treatment is provided. In the second, a specific external cuing device is used to improve gait.

Active Cancellation of Tremor Device

The development of technologies that counter specific symptoms of PD, although not a cure, help to improve the quality of life of those affected. Tremor is one debilitating motor symptom of PD that affects daily activities. Tremor oscillates at a specific frequency range of 2–15 Hz, which can be measured using inertial sensors [61, 62]. The lower frequencies are indicative of a more severe tremor, whereas higher frequencies relate to mild tremor. The ability to measure the degree of tremor has led to the development of tremor cancellation devices. These devices measure the directionality of the tremor and move in the opposite direction to stabilize it.

Pathak et al. [62] designed a spoon that counteracts tremor in the hand, improving utensil accuracy for individuals with mild to moderate tremor (Fig. 10.7b). The

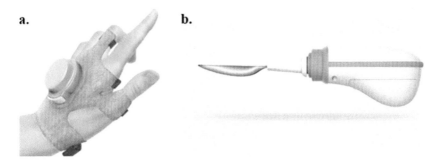

Fig. 10.7 Examples of assistive tremor cancelling devices. (**a**) The GyroGlove™ is worn to reduce hand tremor when the patient requires accurate hand movements, image provided courtesy of GyroGear. (**b**) LiftLabs™ tremor cancelling spoon, which improves accuracy by opposing tremor caused by disease, reproduced with permission from Kozovski [64]

study examined 15 participants diagnosed with essential tremor. The handheld device significantly reduced spoon tremor rated by the UPDRS and accelerometer data [62]. The main strength of this device is the non-invasive nature of the intervention; it is comfortable and easily adopted by its users. However, this device has not proven useful for individuals with severe tremor [62].

The GyroGlove™ is a new technology developed by Faii Ong that reduces tremor continuously (Fig. 10.7a) [63]. The glove is in development with a patent pending, but has the potential to reduce hand tremor in individuals with PD throughout the day. The glove makes use of gyroscopes that resist hand movement and thereby reduce tremors. However, tremor is often multijointed and involves the elbow and shoulder as well.

Laser Cane

Freezing of gait (FOG) is a common symptom in individuals with PD that shows little or no response to pharmacological and surgical interventions [65]. FOG has been estimated to affect 32 % of all individuals diagnosed with PD [66]. Several auditory and visual cues have been used to counter FOG episodes in individuals with PD. Several studies have demonstrated that when PD participants walk across parallel lines on the floor there is an improvement in their FOG episodes [67–69].

The U-Step Laser Cane™ is a walking aid that projects a red laser line across the walking path, making use of the parallel line visual cue (Fig. 10.8). Donovan et al. [70] used the Laser Cane in a population of 26 individuals with PD and found a significant improvement in FOG after 1 month of usage. McCandless et al. [71] compared the Laser Cane with several other auditory and visual cueing interventions in a population of 20 individuals with PD. The Laser Cane was found to be the most effective cueing intervention for correcting FOG episodes [71].

In summary, disability-based rehabilitative approaches:

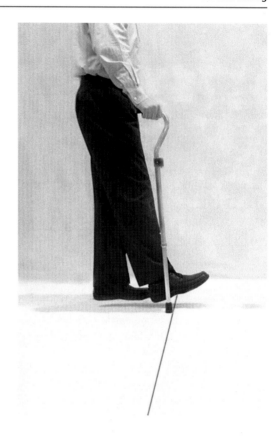

Fig. 10.8 The Laser Cane™ from U-Step™ is used to correct freezing of gait episodes by use of an external laser line cue, image provided courtesy of U-Step

1. Are able to provide patients with temporary relief of the specific motor symptoms that they may be experiencing.
2. Require continual battery replacements and may leave the patient without treatment if replacements are not kept ready.
3. Are adjunctive therapies to medical intervention and may not provide benefit to every patient.
4. Are affordable assistive devices, which makes the use of them possible in patients needing adjunctive symptom relief.

Future Technology-Based Rehabilitation of Parkinson's Disease

Technology will play an increasingly important role in the assessment and in the treatment of MDs. As discussed above, inertial sensors are currently providing real-time feedback on various PD symptoms, allowing treatment regimens to be individualized more efficiently. Physical therapy is also an important factor for the management of PD progression. Physical therapy techniques help to maintain mobility in addition to the treatment provided. As previously discussed, current

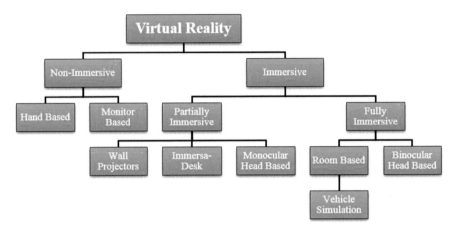

Fig. 10.9   A simplified taxonomy of virtual reality systems

physical therapy techniques are suitable for individuals not diagnosed with PD, use irrelevant tasks, and are performed in contrived spaces. These factors may contribute to the ineffectiveness of these programs in managing motor dysfunction in the PD population. Construction of ecologically valid situations is a necessity when attempting physical therapy for individuals with PD.

As discussed through the chapter, we have now reached a point where the ability to objectively assess the physical disability in the patient can now be supported using a variety of technologies. However, the questions that remain are:

1. How do we carry out these assessments in what would be termed "ecologically valid" environments?
2. How do we provide rehabilitation that then helps patients to optimize their performance within these and the many other environments that we face in our daily life?

Virtual Reality

Virtual reality (VR) may be an optimal tool for a more individualized rehabilitation strategy for individuals with PD. VR is the interaction of an individual in the real world with a virtual environment, which has been generated by a computer. VR can be non-immersive or immersive depending on the technology used (Fig. 10.9). VR makes use of visual, auditory, and haptic inputs, and the virtual environment provides feedback about performance. VR allows an individual to safely explore their environment independently. This technology would provide a flexible and scalable means of implementing realistic and functionally relevant tasks. VR is able to simulate realistic environments that would be too expensive and time-consuming to recreate in the real world for assessment and rehabilitation purposes. VR would address the concern of current research studies that lack contextually relevant stimuli, making generalizability difficult.

1. **Non-immersive VR**: is generally screen-based and pointer-driven. This type of system requires the use of hand-held devices (cell phones, portable games consoles) and monitors (desktop computers).
2. **Partially-immersive VR**: provides the user with an augmentation of the real environment within a virtual environment.
3. **Fully-immersive VR**: provides users with three-dimensional virtual scenes.

Fully immersive VR allows natural interactive behaviors to take place while physiological measures are taken such as body segment movements or brain activity. This allows researchers to address several questions in a controlled environment while recreating real world situations. Furthermore, a fully immersive VR system would engage the sensorimotor system more fully than a simple stimulus, increasing the psychological and behavioral responses. For example, gait difficulty is a major concern in PD as it tends to worsen as the disease progresses. Fully immersive VR allows motor activation to occur during the simulated experience as these environments can allow patients to navigate and physically interact with virtual objects. Fully immersive VR allows the researcher to present multiple stimuli at one time that may not be present in a natural environment. Furthermore, changes can be made to these stimuli at short notice.

Nintendo Wii for Rehabilitation in PD

A recent study examined the use of the Nintendo Wii™ for non-immersive VR rehabilitation in a PD population. The Nintendo Wii is a force platform that provides information on force distribution and center of gravity (Fig. 10.10) [72]. Dos Santos Mendes et al. [72] recruited 16 individuals with PD and 11 controls for the 7-week study. Each participant completed ten training games at each visit. They found that the ability of PD participants to learn, retain, and transfer performance improvements depends on the demands, specifically cognitive demands [72]. It was noted that PD participants were able to transfer motor ability to similar untrained tasks [72].

Gonçalves et al. [73] tested the effectiveness of the Nintendo Wii for VR rehabilitation in 15 individuals with PD. Each training session lasted 40 min, occurring twice a week for 14 sessions. They found a significant improvement on the UPDRS, an increase in walking velocity, and a reduced number of steps during walking [73]. There was no follow-up with patients in the study; the assessments were conducted before training and immediately following training. Moreover, this study failed to demonstrate the appropriate retention of motor training, which is an important factor in physical rehabilitation techniques.

The use of the Nintendo Wii has demonstrated potential therapeutic advantage with rehabilitation in individuals diagnosed with PD. The Nintendo Wii is

Fig. 10.10 The Nintendo Wii™ balance platform used for rehabilitation in PD, image from Wikimedia commons [74]

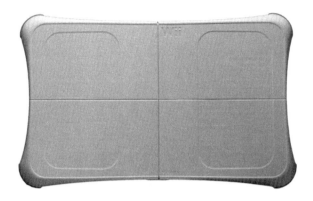

cost-effective, easy to use, and extremely portable. The potential for at-home use is of great advantage with this non-immersive VR device. The drawback is that it is stationary and does not allow patients to be ambulatory during training. Gait training is an important aspect to physical therapy from which individuals with PD would benefit.

Immersive Virtual Reality for Rehabilitation in PD

Research into the implementation of immersive VR for rehabilitation in PD is limited, only appearing in a few published studies. Mirelman et al. [75] developed an immersive VR environment for gait training on a treadmill. Twenty individuals with PD were required and instructed to avoid obstacles in the VR environment while walking on the treadmill. The study lasted 6 weeks and the environment became more challenging as the study progressed to increase adaptability in the participants. Following the 6-week study it was noted that the participants had a significantly improved UPDRS score, gait speed, and stride length [75]. These improvement effects were maintained for up to 4 weeks post-training, and a few metrics continued to improve [75]. This study has several limitations that should be mentioned. The sample size and lack of a control group lower the impact of this study. The ability to compare the training with a control group would rule out any potential placebo or Hawthorne effect. Most importantly, improvement was observed and recorded while on the treadmill only, which lacks ecological validity. Participants must be able to ambulate and practice movement strategies in more realistic VR environments.

Arias et al. [76] tested the validity of using fully immersive VR and virtual environments for assessing PD motor symptoms in ten PD participants. Participants were trained to perform a finger-tapping task in the real environment followed by a virtual environment. An intra-class correlation and the mean difference between the real and virtual finger-tapping test showed high reliability [76]. Immersive VR is in its infancy and has limited implications for PD. Only a few studies have tested the

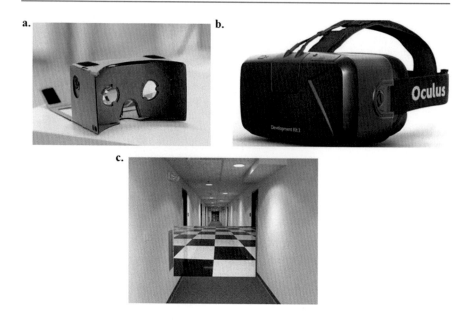

Fig. 10.11 Examples of virtual reality devices and a scenario. (a) The Google™ cardboard goggles provide an affordable alternative to virtual reality glasses using a smart phone, image from Wikimedia commons [78]. (b) Oculus Rift™ virtual reality headset, image from flickr creative commons [79]. (c) An augmented virtual reality scenario for freezing of gait in PD, reproduced with permission from Holmes [80]

application in a population of individuals with PD. Furthermore, the cost of these devices is currently fairly high, making personal use unfeasible. However, immersive VR is a promising rehabilitation technique that can provide a controlled, comfortable environment in which patients can complete ecologically valid tasks.

Augmented Immersive Virtual Reality Assessment and Treatment

Augmented immersive VR is the visual combination of the real-world environment with computer generated imagery (Fig. 10.11c) [77]. Instead of being immersed in a complete virtually simulated world, augmented reality allows the subject to experience a different location while staying connected with reality [77]. This form of VR allows for a more realistic virtual environment through which subjects can navigate. A recent augmented VR method has been established for individuals diagnosed with PD. Garcia et al. [77] proposed a method by which patients experience ecologically valid scenarios to navigate. The three scenarios that were established in augmented reality were watering plants, shopping in a grocery store, and crossing a busy street [77]. These scenarios were chosen as real-world situations in which individuals with PD would find themselves.

The preliminary work clearly shows that it is now possible to design and construct scenarios that allow the assessment of patients with disorders such as PD within contextually relevant environments. This can be carried out using portable VR devices (Oculus Rift™, Google™ VR goggles, etc.) within a reasonable amount of space (Fig. 10.11a, b). Scenarios can be built to meet the major disability for the patient and implemented in their area of residence. Based upon the deficits elicited, a program can be designed, again in the same immersive environment, to provide rehabilitation to these patients with interesting, increasingly complex environments.

Conclusion

When discussing the future perspective of complete care for individuals with PD it is important to consider assessment methods, treatment techniques, and rehabilitation strategies. It is clear that technology will play an important role in the future of PD and other MDs in general. The ability to assess and monitor motor symptoms objectively and quantitatively with technology is reaching a state of maturity where portable, cost-effective methodologies are now becoming available. This will allow current treatments to be better targeted for each individual and more accurately test the efficacy of new treatments. Rehabilitation is a feasible adjunctive therapy for PD that maximizes the functional ability of each patient according to their disease state. Developing a program that employs ecologically valid scenarios in a comfortable environment for assessment will greatly enhance the effectiveness of the technique. When combined with objective measurement tools, the assessment of patient deficits in active scenario-based settings can provide a true picture of the real-world disabilities faced by patients in daily life. The same techniques can then be employed to generate a rehabilitative program that is individualized and targeted. The future of PD care relies on such individualized and optimized treatment and rehabilitation techniques that make use of advancing technology.

References

1. Yang K, Xiong WX, Liu FT, Sun YM, Luo S, Ding ZT, et al. Objective and quantitative assessment of motor function in Parkinson's disease from the perspective of practical applications [Internet]. Ann Transl Med. 2016;4(5):90. http://atm.amegroups.com/article/view/9420/10095.
2. Heldman DA, Giuffrida JP, Chen R, Payne M, Mazzella F, Duker AP, et al. The modified bradykinesia rating scale for Parkinson's disease: reliability and comparison with kinematic measures [Internet]. Mov Disord. 2011;26(10):1859–63. http://www.ncbi.nlm.nih.gov/pubmed/21538531.
3. Mera TO, Heldman DA, Espay AJ, Payne M, Giuffrida JP. Feasibility of home-based automated Parkinson's disease motor assessment [Internet]. J Neurosci Methods. 2012;203(1):152–6. http://www.ncbi.nlm.nih.gov/pubmed/21978487.
4. Egerton T, Thingstad P, Helbostad JL. Comparison of programs for determining temporal-spatial gait variables from instrumented walkway data: PKmas versus GAITRite [Internet]. BMC Res Notes. 2014;7(1):542. http://www.ncbi.nlm.nih.gov/pubmed/25134621.
5. Pahwa R, Lyons KE. Early diagnosis of Parkinson's disease: recommendations from diagnostic clinical guidelines [Internet]. Am J Manag Care. 2010;16(Suppl I):S94–9. http://www.ncbi.nlm.nih.gov/pubmed/20297872.
6. Burke RE, O'Malley K. Axon degeneration in Parkinson's disease [Internet]. Exp Neurol. 2013;246:72–83. doi:10.1016/j.expneurol.2012.01.011.

7. Gunn DG, Naismith SL, Lewis SJG. Sleep disturbances in Parkinson disease and their potential role in heterogeneity [Internet]. J Geriatr Psychiatry Neurol. 2010;23(2):131–7. http://www.ncbi.nlm.nih.gov/pubmed/20101072.

8. Lindgren HS, Dunnett SB. Cognitive dysfunction and depression in Parkinson's disease: what can be learned from rodent models? [Internet]. Eur J Neurosci. 2012;35(12):1894–907. doi:10.1111/j.1460-9568.2012.08162.x.

9. Bonnet AM, Jutras MF, Czernecki V, Corvol JC, Vidailhet M. Nonmotor symptoms in Parkinson's disease in 2012: relevant clinical aspects [Internet]. Parkinson's Dis. 2012;2012:198316. doi:10.1155/2012/198316.

10. Chien S-L, Lin S-Z, Liang C-C, Soong Y-S, Lin S-H, Hsin Y-L, et al. The efficacy of quantitative gait analysis by the GAITRite system in evaluation of parkinsonian bradykinesia [Internet]. Parkinsonism Relat Disord. 2006;12(7):438–42. http://www.ncbi.nlm.nih.gov/pubmed/16798053.

11. Clark EC, Clements BG, Erickson DJ, Maccarty CS, Mulder DW. Therapeutic exercises in management of paralysis agitans [Internet]. J Am Med Assoc. 1956;162(11):1041–3. http://www.ncbi.nlm.nih.gov/pubmed/13366704.

12. Birkmayer W, Hornykiewicz O. Der L-dioxyphenylalanin (=L-DOPA)-Effekt beim Parkinson-Syndrom des <enschen: zur Pathogenese und Behandlung der Parkinson-Akinese [Internet]. Arch Psychiat Nervenkr. 1962;203(5):560–74. doi:10.1007/BF00343235.

13. Tomlinson CL, Patel S, Meek C, Clarke CE, Stowe R, Shah L, et al. Physiotherapy versus placebo or no intervention in Parkinson's disease [Internet]. Cochrane Database Syst Rev. 2012;7(8), CD002817. http://www.ncbi.nlm.nih.gov/pubmed/22786482.

14. Clarke CE, Patel S, Ives N, Rick CE, Dowling F, Woolley R, et al. Physiotherapy and occupational therapy vs no therapy in mild to moderate Parkinson disease: a randomized clinical trial [Internet]. JAMA Neurol. 2016;73(3):291–9. http://www.ncbi.nlm.nih.gov/pubmed/26785394.

15. Goetz CG, Tilley BC, Shaftman SR, Stebbins GT, Fahn S, Martinez-Martin P, et al. Movement disorder society-sponsored revision of the unified Parkinson's disease rating scale (MDS-UPDRS): scale presentation and clinimetric testing results [Internet]. Mov Disord. 2008;23(15):2129–70. doi:10.1002/mds.22340.

16. Windolf M, Götzen N, Morlock M. Systematic accuracy and precision analysis of video motion capturing systems—exemplified on the Vicon-460 system [Internet]. J Biomech. 2008;41(12):2776–80. http://search.proquest.com/docview/1651859645?accountid=12347\n; http://sfx.scholarsportal.info/mcmaster?url_ver=Z39.88-2004&rft_val_fmt=info:ofi/fmt:kev:mtx:journal&genre=article&sid=ProQ:ProQ:ericshell&atitle=Classroom-Based+Narrative+and+Vocabulary+Inst.

17. Galna B, Barry G, Jackson D, Mhiripiri D, Olivier P, Rochester L. Accuracy of the Microsoft Kinect sensor for measuring movement in people with Parkinson's disease [Internet]. Gait Posture. 2014;39(4):1062–8. doi:10.1016/j.gaitpost.2014.01.008.

18. Das S, Trutoiu L, Murai A, Alcindor D, Oh M, De la Torre F, et al. Quantitative measurement of motor symptoms in Parkinson's disease: a study with full-body motion capture data [Internet]. Conf Proc IEEE Eng Med Biol Soc. 2011;2011:6789–92. http://www.ncbi.nlm.nih.gov/pubmed/22255897.

19. Mirek E, Rudzińska M, Szczudlik A. The assessment of gait disorders in patients with Parkinson's disease using the three-dimensional motion analysis system Vicon [Internet]. Neurol Neurochir Pol. 2007;41(2):128–33. http://www.ncbi.nlm.nih.gov/pubmed/17530574.

20. MocapHouse. Motion capture systems managed by IT backyard [Internet]. Introduction to Vicon F40 Camera; 2010. http://www.mocaphouse.com/"http://www.mocaphouse.com/, http://itbackyard.com/mocaphouse"http://itbackyard.com/mocaphouse

21. Bilney B, Morris M, Webster K. Concurrent related validity of the GAITRite walkway system for quantification of the spatial and temporal parameters of gait [Internet]. Gait Posture. 2003;17(1):68–74. http://linkinghub.elsevier.com/retrieve/pii/S096663620200053X.

22. Menz HB, Latt MD, Tiedemann A, Mun San Kwan M, Lord SR. Reliability of the GAITRite walkway system for the quantification of temporo-spatial parameters of gait in young and older people [Internet]. Gait Posture. 2004;20(1):20–5. http://www.ncbi.nlm.nih.gov/pubmed/15196515.

23. McDonough AL, Batavia M, Chen FC, Kwon S, Ziai J. The validity and reliability of the GAITRite system's measurements: a preliminary evaluation [Internet]. Arch Phys Med Rehabil. 2001;82(3):419–25. http://www.ncbi.nlm.nih.gov/pubmed/11245768.
24. van Uden CJT, Besser MP. Test-retest reliability of temporal and spatial gait characteristics measured with an instrumented walkway system (GAITRite) [Internet]. BMC Musculoskelet Disord. 2004;5(13):13. http://www.ncbi.nlm.nih.gov/pubmed/15147583.
25. Egerton T, Williams DR, Iansek R. Comparison of gait in progressive supranuclear palsy, Parkinson's disease and healthy older adults [Internet]. BMC Neurol. 2012;12(1):116. http://www.ncbi.nlm.nih.gov/pubmed/23031506.
26. Lord S, Galna B, Coleman S, Burn D, Rochester L. Mild depressive symptoms are associated with gait impairment in early Parkinson's disease [Internet]. Mov Disord. 2013;28(5):634–9. http://www.ncbi.nlm.nih.gov/pubmed/23390120.
27. Verghese J, Holtzer R, Lipton RB, Wang C. Quantitative gait markers and incident fall risk in older adults [Internet]. J Gerontol A Biol Sci Med Sci. 2009;64(8):896–901. doi:10.1093/gerona/glp033.
28. Hass CJ, Malczak P, Nocera J, Stegemöller EL, Shukala A, Malaty I, et al. Quantitative normative Gait data in a large cohort of ambulatory persons with Parkinson's disease [Internet]. PLoS One. 2012;7(8), e42337. http://www.ncbi.nlm.nih.gov/pmc/articles/PMC3411737/.
29. Robles-García V, Corral-Bergantiños Y, Espinosa N, Jácome MA, García-Sancho C, Cudeiro J, et al. Spatiotemporal gait patterns during overt and covert evaluation in patients with Parkinson's disease and healthy subjects: is there a Hawthorne effect? [Internet]. J Appl Biomech. 2015;31(3):189–94.
30. Patel S, Chen BR, Buckley T, Rednic R, McClure D, Tarsy D, et al. Home monitoring of patients with Parkinson's disease via wearable technology and a web-based application [Internet]. Conf Proc IEEE Eng Med Biol Soc. 2010;2010:4411–14. http://www.ncbi.nlm.nih.gov/pubmed/21096462.
31. Cancela J, Arredondo MT, Hurtado O. Proposal of a Kinect(TM)-based system for gait assessment and rehabilitation in Parkinson's disease [Internet]. Conf Proc IEEE Eng Med Biol Soc. 2014;2014:4519–22. http://www.ncbi.nlm.nih.gov/pubmed/25570996.
32. Wikimedia. Xbox Kinect Sensor [Internet]. 2014. p. Xbox-One-Kinect. https://commons.wikimedia.org/wiki/File:Xbox-One-Kinect.jpg.
33. Geerse DJ, Coolen BH, Roerdink M. Kinematic validation of a multi-kinect v2 instrumented 10-meter walkway for quantitative gait assessments [Internet]. PLoS One. 2015;10(10), e0139913. http://www.ncbi.nlm.nih.gov/pubmed/26461498.
34. Dobkin BH. Wearable motion sensors to continuously measure real-world physical activities [Internet]. Curr Opin Neurol. 2013;26(6):602–8. http://ec.europa.eu/public_opinion/archives/ebs/ebs_183_6_en.pdf.
35. Cuesta-Vargas AI, Galán-Mercant A, Williams JM. The use of inertial sensors system for human motion analysis [Internet]. Phys Ther Rev. 2010;15(6):462–73. doi:10.1179/1743288X11Y.0000000006.
36. Rahimi F, Duval C, Jog M, Bee C, South A, Jog M, et al. Capturing whole-body mobility of patients with Parkinson disease using inertial motion sensors: expected challenges and rewards [Internet]. Conf Proc IEEE Eng Med Biol Soc. 2011;2011:5833–8. http://www.ncbi.nlm.nih.gov/pubmed/22255666.
37. Rahimi F, Bee C, Duval C, Boissy P, Edwards R, Jog M, et al. Using ecological whole body kinematics to evaluate effects of medication adjustment in Parkinson disease [Internet]. J Parkinson's Dis. 2014;4(4):617–27. http://www.ncbi.nlm.nih.gov/pubmed/25055960.
38. Tao W, Liu T, Zheng R, Feng H. Gait analysis using wearable sensors [Internet]. Sensors. 2012;12(12):2255–83. http://www.mdpi.com/1424-8220/12/2/2255/.
39. Chang SY, Lai CF, Chao HCJ, Park JH, Huang YM. An environmental-adaptive fall detection system on mobile device [Internet]. J Med Syst. 2011;35(5):1299–312. http://www.ncbi.nlm.nih.gov/pubmed/21424848.

40. Sant'Anna A, Salarian A, Wickström N. A new measure of movement symmetry in early Parkinson's disease patients using symbolic processing of inertial sensor data [Internet]. IEEE Trans Biomed Eng. 2011;58(7):2127–35. http://www.ncbi.nlm.nih.gov/pubmed/21536527.

41. Salarian A, Russmann H, Vingerhoets FJG, Burkhard PR, Aminian K. Ambulatory monitoring of physical activities in patients with Parkinson's disease [Internet]. IEEE Trans Biomed Eng. 2007;54(12):2296–9. http://ieeexplore.ieee.org/stamp/stamp.jsp?arnumber=04359998.

42. Ahlskog JE, Uitti RJ. Rasagiline, Parkinson neuroprotection, and delayed-start trials: still no satisfaction? [Internet]. Neurology. 2010;74(14):1143–8. http://www.ncbi.nlm.nih.gov/pubmed/20368634.

43. Giuffrida JP, Riley DE, Maddux BN, Heldman DA. Clinically deployable Kinesia™ technology for automated tremor assessment [Internet]. Mov Disord. 2009;24(5):723–30. http://resolver.scholarsportal.info/resolve/08853185/v24i0005/723_cdktfata.

44. Heldman DA, Espay AJ, LeWitt PA, Giuffrida JP. Clinician versus machine: reliability and responsiveness of motor endpoints in Parkinson's disease [Internet]. Parkinsonism Relat Disord. 2014;20(6):590–5. http://www.ncbi.nlm.nih.gov/pubmed/24661464.

45. Marinus J, van Hilten JJ. The significance of motor (a)symmetry in Parkinson's disease [Internet]. Mov Disord. 2015;30(3):379–85. http://www.ncbi.nlm.nih.gov/pubmed/25546239.

46. Hoehn MM, Yahr MD. Parkinsonism: onset, progression and mortality [Internet]. Neurology. 1967;17(5):427–42. http://www.ncbi.nlm.nih.gov/pubmed/6067254.

47. Cutti AG, Giovanardi A, Rocchi L, Davalli A. A simple test to assess the static and dynamic accuracy of an inertial sensors system for human movement analysis [Internet]. Conf Proc IEEE Eng Med Biol Soc. 2006;1:5912–15. http://www.ncbi.nlm.nih.gov/pubmed/17946728.

48. Nguyen HP, Ayachi F, Lavigne-Pelletier C, Blamoutier M, Rahimi F, Boissy P, et al. Auto detection and segmentation of physical activities during a Timed-Up-and-Go (TUG) task in healthy older adults using multiple inertial sensors [Internet]. J Neuroeng Rehabil. 2015;12:36. http://www.ncbi.nlm.nih.gov/pubmed/25885438.

49. LHSC. LHSC Inside Magazine [Internet]. London, Canada. 2015. p. The Movement Towards BetterTreatmentofParkinson.http://inside.lhsc.on.ca/article/summer-2015/movement-towards-better-treatment-parkinsons.

50. Nijkrake MJ, Keus SHJ, Kalf JG, Sturkenboom IHWM, Munneke M, Kappellea C, et al. Allied health care interventions and complementary therapies in Parkinson's disease [Internet]. Parkinsonism Relat Disord. 2007;13 Suppl 3:S488–94. http://www.ncbi.nlm.nih.gov/pubmed/18267288.

51. Rubenis J. A rehabilitational approach to the management of Parkinson's disease [Internet]. Parkinsonism Relat Disord. 2007;13 Suppl 3:S495–7. http://www.ncbi.nlm.nih.gov/pubmed/18267289.

52. Keus SHJ, Munneke M, Nijkrake MJ, Kwakkel G, Bloem BR. Physical therapy in Parkinson's disease: evolution and future challenges [Internet]. Mov Disord. 2009;24(1):1–14. http://www.ncbi.nlm.nih.gov/pubmed/18946880.

53. Morris ME. Movement disorders in people with Parkinson disease: a model for physical therapy [Internet]. Phys Ther. 2000;80(6):578–97. http://www.ncbi.nlm.nih.gov/pubmed/10842411.

54. Debaere F, Wenderoth N, Sunaert S, Van Hecke P, Swinnen SP. Internal vs external generation of movements: differential neural pathways involved in bimanual coordination performed in the presence or absence of augmented visual feedback [Internet]. Neuroimage. 2003;19(3):764–76. http://www.ncbi.nlm.nih.gov/pubmed/12880805.

55. Goldberg G. Supplementary motor area structure and function: review and hypotheses [Internet]. Behav Brain Sci. 1985;8(04):567. http://www.journals.cambridge.org/abstract_S0140525X00045167.

56. Verschueren SM, Swinnen SPP, Dom R, De Weerdt W. Interlimb coordination in patients with Parkinson's disease: motor learning deficits and the importance of augmented information feedback [Internet]. Exp Brain Res. 1997;113(3):497–508. http://www.ncbi.nlm.nih.gov/pubmed/9108216.

57. Samuel M, Ceballos-Baumann AO, Blin J, Uema T, Boecker H, Passingham RE, et al. Evidence for lateral premotor and parietal overactivity in Parkinson's disease during sequential

and bimanual movements. A PET study [Internet]. Brain. 1997;120(Pt 6):963–76. http://www. ncbi.nlm.nih.gov/pubmed/9217681.

58. Hackney ME, Lee HL, Battisto J, Crosson B, McGregor KM. Context-dependent neural activation: internally and externally guided rhythmic lower limb movement in individuals with and without neurodegenerative disease [Internet]. Front Neurol. 2015;6(6):251. doi:10.3389/fneur.2015.00251.

59. Morris ME. Locomotor training in people with Parkinson disease [Internet]. Phys Ther. 2006;86(10):1426–35. http://www.ncbi.nlm.nih.gov/pubmed/17012646.

60. King LA, Horak FB. Delaying mobility disability in people with Parkinson disease using a sensorimotor agility exercise program [Internet]. Phys Ther. 2009;89(4):384–93. http://www. ncbi.nlm.nih.gov/pubmed/19228832.

61. Calzetti S, Baratti M, Gresty M, Findley L. Frequency/amplitude characteristics of postural tremor of the hands in a population of patients with bilateral essential tremor: implications for the classification and mechanism of essential tremor [Internet]. J Neurol Neurosurg Psychiatry. 1987;50(5):561–7. http://www.ncbi.nlm.nih.gov/pubmed/3585381.

62. Pathak A, Redmond JA, Allen M, Chou KL. A noninvasive handheld assistive device to accommodate essential tremor: a pilot study [Internet]. Mov Disord. 2014;29(6):838–42. http://www.ncbi.nlm.nih.gov/pubmed/24375570.

63. Parkin S. MIT Technology Review [Internet]. 2016. p. Hope in a Glove for Parkinson's Patients. https://www.technologyreview.com/s/545456/hope-in-a-glove-for-parkinsons-patients/.

64. Kozovski A. RateMDs: Doctors Reviews and Ratings [Internet]. 2016. p. This Smart Spoon AidsParkinson'sPatientsinFeed.https://www.ratemds.com/blog/this-smart-spoon-aids-parkinsons-patients-in-feeding-themselves/.

65. Nonnekes J, Snijders AH, Nutt JG, Deuschl G, Giladi N, Bloem BR. Freezing of gait: a practical approach to management [Internet]. Lancet Neurol. 2015;14(7):768–78. http://www.ncbi. nlm.nih.gov/pubmed/26018593.

66. Giladi N, McMahon D, Przedborski S, Flaster E, Guillory S, Kostic V, et al. Motor blocks in Parkinson's disease [Internet]. Neurology. 1992;42(2):333–9. http://www.ncbi.nlm.nih.gov/pubmed/1736161.

67. Azulay JP, Mesure S, Amblard B, Blin O, Sangla I, Pouget J. Visual control of locomotion in Parkinson's disease [Internet]. Brain. 1999;122(Pt 1):111–20. http://www.ncbi.nlm.nih.gov/pubmed/10050899.

68. Suteerawattananon M, Morris GS, Etnyre BR, Jankovic J, Protas EJ. Effects of visual and auditory cues on gait in individuals with Parkinson's disease [Internet]. J Neurol Sci. 2004;219(1–2):63–9. http://www.ncbi.nlm.nih.gov/pubmed/15050439.

69. Jiang Y, Norman KE. Effects of visual and auditory cues on gait initiation in people with Parkinson's disease [Internet]. Clin Rehabil. 2006;20(1):36–45. http://www.ncbi.nlm.nih.gov/pubmed/16502748.

70. Donovan S, Lim C, Diaz N, Browner N, Rose P, Sudarsky LR, et al. Laserlight cues for gait freezing in Parkinson's disease: an open-label study [Internet]. Parkinsonism Relat Disord. 2011;17(4):240–5. doi:10.1016/j.parkreldis.2010.08.010.

71. McCandless PJ, Evans BJ, Janssen J, Selfe J, Churchill A, Richards J. Effect of three cueing devices for people with Parkinson's disease with gait initiation difficulties [Internet]. Gait Posture. 2016;44:7–11. http://www.sciencedirect.com/science/article/pii/S096663621500942X.

72. dos Santos Mendes FA, Pompeu JE, Modenesi Lobo A, Guedes da Silva K, Oliveira T de P, Peterson Zomignani A, et al. Motor learning, retention and transfer after virtual-reality-based training in Parkinson's disease--effect of motor and cognitive demands of games: a longitudinal, controlled clinical study [Internet]. Physiotherapy. 2012;98(3):217–23. doi:10.1016/j.physio.2012.06.001.

73. Gonçalves GB, Leite MAA, Orsini M, Pereira JS. Effects of using the Nintendo wii fit plus platform in the sensorimotor training of gait disorders in Parkinson's disease [Internet]. Neurol Int. 2014;6(1):5048. http://www.ncbi.nlm.nih.gov/pubmed/24744845.

74. Wikimedia. Wii Balance Board [Internet]. 2011. p. Wii Balance Board for Nintendi Wii. https://commons.wikimedia.org/wiki/File:Wii_Balance_Board_transparent.png.

75. Mirelman A, Maidan I, Herman T, Deutsch JE, Giladi N, Hausdorff JM. Virtual reality for gait training: can it induce motor learning to enhance complex walking and reduce fall risk in patients with Parkinson's disease? [Internet]. J Gerontol A Biol Sci Med Sci. 2011;66(2):234–40. http://www.ncbi.nlm.nih.gov/pubmed/21106702.
76. Arias P, Robles-García V, Sanmartín G, Flores J, Cudeiro J. Virtual reality as a tool for evaluation of repetitive rhythmic movements in the elderly and Parkinson's disease patients [Internet]. PLoS One. 2012;7(1), e30021. http://www.ncbi.nlm.nih.gov/pubmed/22279559.
77. Garcia A, Andre N, Bell Boucher D, Roberts-South A, Jog M, Katchabaw M. Immersive augmented reality for Parkinson disease rehabilitation. In: Intelligent systems reference library [Internet]. Berlin: Springer; 2014. p. 445–69. http://www.scopus.com/inward/record.url?eid=2-s2.0-84927509975&partnerID=tZOtx3y1.
78. Wikimedia. Google cardboard VR mount [Internet]. 2014. p. Assembled Google cardboard VRmount. https://commons.wikimedia.org/wiki/File:Assembled_Google_Cardboard_VR_mount.jpg.
79. DiCarlo, Eleni. Oculus Rift [Internet]. 2014. Flikr. New Oculus Rift Now Available for Developers. https://www.flickr.com/photos/bagogames/13300603614.
80. Holmes A. Online Press Release Distribution Service [Internet]. Palm Springs. 2010. p. Parkinson's Gait Dramatically Improves with High Tech Visual Feedback Device. http://ww1.prweb.com/prfiles/2010/04/11/689374/GaitAidsuperimp.jpg.

Index

© Springer International Publishing Switzerland 2017   183
H.F. Chien, O.G.P. Barsottini (eds.), *Movement Disorders Rehabilitation*,
DOI 10.1007/978-3-319-46062-8

Printed in the United States
By Bookmasters